Book index

Introduction to the book

Medicinal plants heal or help recovery

Medicinal plants contribute to the healing process or to the alleviation of various diseases. Let's learn about its advantages, side effects, and ways to use it. In a series of alternative medicine books

The plants we know, whether those found in pots, in the garden or in the courtyard of the house. Its benefits are not limited to decoration only. As is known, plants have another important role in our lives. Since ancient times, they have played a role in treating us. That's why medicinal plants as we know them exist.

Since the Middle Ages, man has believed that there are medicinal herbs that can cure him. Also today, in the era of synthetic medicines, people believe that medicinal plants have the ability to help them recover from various diseases. People who have been treated with naturopathy, a treatment in which a person heals himself using various methods, are accustomed to using medicinal herbs as part of the treatment, along with those methods that he uses to heal himself.

Medicinal herbs can help in many cases, whether in the healing process or in alleviating various diseases. Of course, every use of medicinal herbs must be carried out according to the type of disease we suffer from. Each plant has a number of features, so there are plants, which can help with several disease conditions. In addition, when we mix several plants together, we lose the qualities of those plants, and we get a mixture of these plants.

Medicinal plants, like regular medicines, also have side effects. Therefore, it is important to examine the dose we take, and how long we should consume this plant. It is important to clarify that medicinal herbs cannot cure diseases such as cancer, heart, or other serious diseases, but only help relieve the pain caused by these diseases. Therefore, it does not come as an alternative to traditional medicines.

Treatment with medicinal plants, of course, is not the only method of treatment. Physiotherapy believes that a person must maintain proper nutrition, regular physical activity, avoid substances dangerous to the body, and avoid stress and various pressures, in order to maintain good health.

Medicinal herbs are not sold today as they were sold in the past. Although different parts of plants are still used, but not in the same way as in the past. Today different concentrations or compounds are used, rather than taking the plants as they are. Any purchase of medicinal plants from a natural products store or pharmacy must be done through consultation with a person specialized in natural herbal medicine. This is after diagnosing the problem we are suffering from. The plant is taken according to its properties, knowing that over time we will have to use other medicinal plants, depending on the course of treatment of the disease.

How to use medicinal plants?

There are different ways to use medicinal plants. Extract, where boiling water is poured over the plant flowers, filtered and drunk. Steeping, where boiling water is poured over a large amount of plant material, and after twenty minutes it is drunk. Boiled, all parts of the plant are boiled with water, here also the solid parts of the plant are used, such as roots, stems, peels and seeds. Ointments, in this case the plant powder is mixed with fat.

Medicinal plants are used, depending on the type of flower and the type of treatment we want to obtain. It is important to clarify that treatment with medical herbs may not be sufficient for recovery. When we notice that the disease has not gone away, we must consult a doctor before it is too late.

All this and more we will learn about in this series. Follow us

Natural medicine is the ability of man to treat himself!

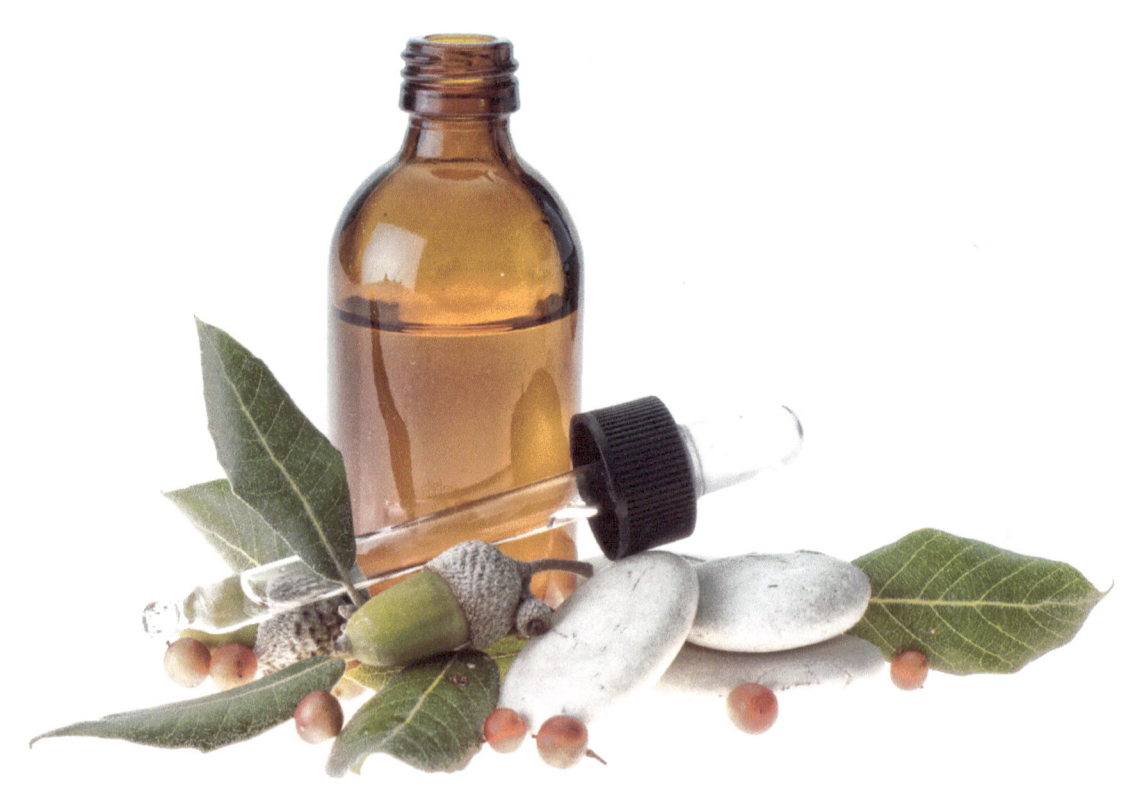

Natural medicine is a group of methods that refer to a person's ability to heal himself through auxiliary means. Including: medicinal herbs, prescription medicine, food additives, physical activity, and others.

Since time immemorial, man has sought in different ways and methods to treat himself from the various medical problems that he suffers from. Even after the emergence of modern medicine that we know, man is still looking for other ways to heal himself. One of the alternative methods found by man is natural healing, that is, self-healing, believing in the human ability to treat himself

Natural medicine methods originated from different streams in alternative medicine , since the eighteenth and nineteenth centuries, when Dr. John Schell developed this concept in 1895. However, the roots of this method can be found in Hippocrates, who opposed the superstitions that people believed in and that It can heal man, as he claimed, unlike them, that only man and nature can heal man.

Natural medicine is a group of methods that believe that a person can heal himself by means of aids. These means can be: medicinal herbs, prescription medication, proper diet, food additives, physical activity and treatment of the sensitive side of the problem. The claim is that by means of these means, a person can avoid and combat the effects of unhealthy food, external infection, lack of physical activity, and others, as these effects lead to a person living in an unhealthy pattern, of course, while natural medicine methods can help influence against These factors to contend with.

Naturopaths claim that since man is part of nature, he can heal himself, as only natural means can heal man. Thus, a person can exploit his natural abilities to heal himself. Nature gives man the necessary support to heal his body, and thus strengthens him. This process is long-term and requires a person to change his behavior and thinking patterns. Thus, he maintains his health, balance and allows him to be protected from external factors that may pose a threat to him.

It is important to note that these aids should only be used as complements and not as main aids. Otherwise, the human body will suffer from deficiency. For example, nutritional supplements do not replace food itself. Physical exercise does not replace a good sleep. In order to conduct effective and sound treatment, the goals that must be achieved and the principles that must be followed must be determined, and then implemented in stages.

It should be noted that there are quite a few criticisms of this method. The main claim is that these aids are not sufficient, and that the majority of patients who are treated in this way still refuse to receive conventional treatment despite their suffering from the disease, which puts them at risk of being too late for them and their chances of recovery.

In order to receive the correct treatment with naturopathy, you should consult a qualified naturopath, get all the necessary information from him, and understand what naturopathy is. In order for the treatment to be successful, it must be performed continuously, diligently and carefully. In cases of illness or severe pain, one must go to the attending physician before the situation deteriorates, because then nothing can be done to save the patient's body, or his psyche in other cases.

Treating colds with herbs

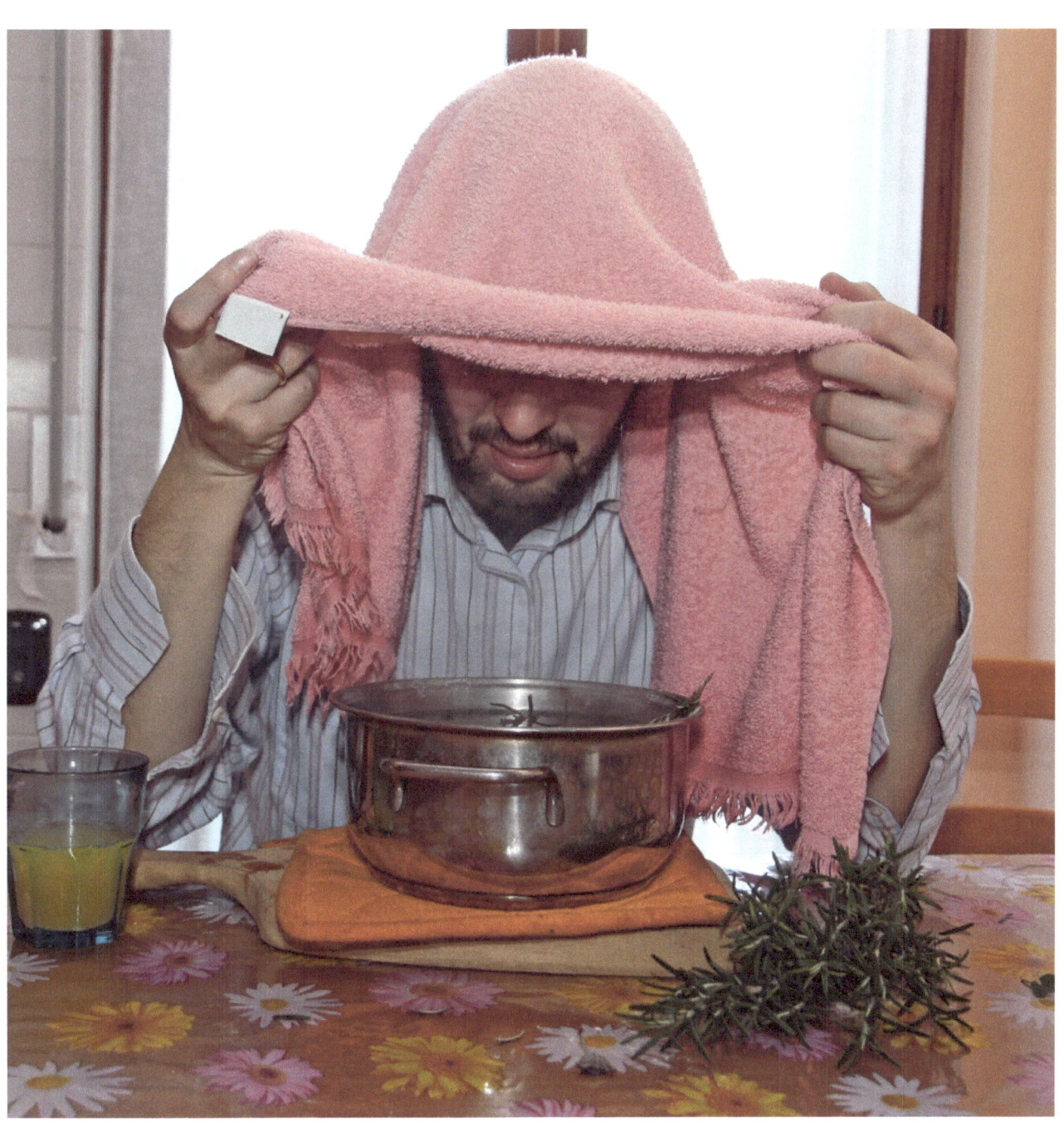

There are many natural methods that claim to be able to treat the common cold, but how are colds treated with herbs?

The common cold is caused by viruses, so antibiotics cannot be used in treatment. However, some herbs can be used to reduce the severity of symptoms associated with a cold or shorten the duration of infection. Below we will learn about some of these herbs:

Treating colds with herbs: What is the truth about this?

There are many herbs that offer potential benefits in treating colds, but you should consult your doctor before using any of these herbs. Among these herbs we mention:

1. Ginger

Ginger is one of the herbal ways to treat colds. Ginger contains many compounds, such as gingerols and shogaols. These compounds provide anti-inflammatory properties that reduce the severity of cold symptoms, such as throat pain and nausea.

Ginger can be used to treat colds by drinking a cup of boiling water containing thin slices of ginger.

2. Astragalus

Astragalus can be used as one of the herbal treatments for colds. Astragalus contains many antioxidant and antiviral properties, and it also works to enhance the immune system's ability to fight various infections.

You can benefit from the benefits of astragalus herb by drinking astragalus tea or consuming nutritional supplements that contain extracts of this herb.

3. Ginseng

Ginseng is one of the herbal ways to treat colds. Because it contains polysaccharide compounds and ginsenosides, which help both reduce the severity of cold symptoms and reduce the duration of colds.

Ginseng can be used to treat colds by eating it in its raw form or drinking ginseng tea.

4. Elderberry

Elderberry contains anthocyanins, which enhance the functioning of the immune system and fight viral infections. Elderberry can be used as a way to treat colds with herbs by eating it alone or using it in dessert dishes.

5. Mint

Mint can be used as a method of treating colds with herbs. Because it contains the compound menthol, which has the ability to fight the pain associated with colds and nasal congestion , which facilitates the breathing process during a cold.

Menthol can be used by inhaling water vapor containing menthol oil or by applying it to the pillow on which the patient sleeps at night.

Treating colds with other natural methods

In addition to methods of treating colds with herbs, there are many other natural methods that help in treatment, such as:

1-Hydration: Moisturizing the body from the inside is one of the important steps in treating colds, as drinking water, juices, and soups helps get rid of nasal congestion.

2-Gargling: Gargling with a saline solution consisting of half a teaspoon of salt dissolved in 240 milliliters of warm water helps get rid of throat pain .

3-Consumption of honey: Honey helps get rid of throat pain, and it can be eaten with a spoon or dissolved in a cup of tea.

4-Citrus consumption: Citrus fruits contain vitamin C, which helps raise the body's immunity and get rid of phlegm. Citrus fruits can be eaten alone or added lemon juice to a cup of warm tea.

When should you visit a doctor?

There are some conditions that may accompany the common cold and require a visit to the doctor. Among these cases we mention:

Symptoms persist for more than 10 days despite using methods of treating colds with herbs and other natural methods.

The presence of chronic diseases that the patient suffers from.

Pregnancy.

Symptoms of the common cold appear in people over the age of 65.

Cold symptoms appear in infants younger than 3 months.

5 herbs to treat irritable bowel syndrome

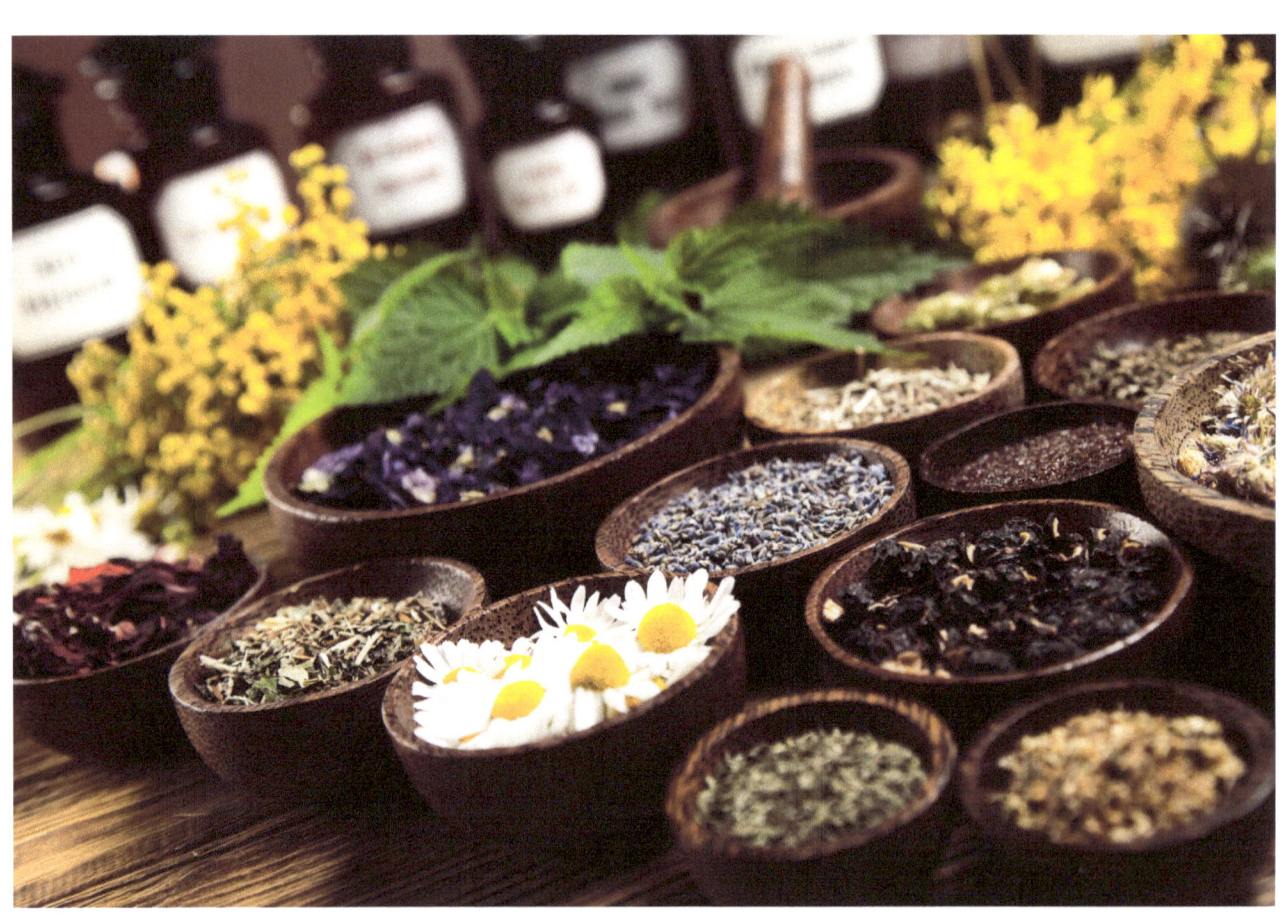

Irritable bowel syndrome is an annoying problem for many. Here we will present to you a group of herbs to treat irritable bowel syndrome.

If you suffer from the problem of irritable bowel syndrome, it may be very useful to drink herbal tea, which will relieve bloating, gas, and the annoying symptoms associated with irritable bowel syndrome. What are the most important herbs for treating irritable bowel syndrome ?

Herbs to treat irritable bowel syndrome

Among the most important and best herbs used to treat irritable bowel syndrome, which are followed by many individuals who suffer from this type of health condition, are the following:

1. Peppermint tea

Mint is one of the most famous herbs for treating the colon and its symptoms as well. It works to relax the digestive system, relax its muscles, and treat its various problems, such as colic, bloating, gas, and intestinal cramps.

It has been shown that the role that mint plays in treating the symptoms of irritable bowel syndrome, as it has been shown to contribute to relaxing the intestinal muscles and is considered a gas repellent, and as for the method of using it, it is done by following the following:

You can boil mint leaves and drink it directly.

Soak mint leaves for a while in lukewarm water; Then drink the infusion.

Add peppermint oil to hot water.

2. Anise tea

Anise has long been used to treat many health problems, especially digestive and stomach problems. It is an herb for the colon. Because it has soothing properties, it is considered one of the best herbs for treating irritable bowel syndrome. As for how to use it, it is done by boiling or soaking a tablespoon of anise seeds in lukewarm water, or adding its powder to two cups of boiling water and drinking it to get the benefit.

2. Anise tea

3. Fennel tea

Fennel tea is a remedy used to expel gas, get rid of bloating and intestinal problems. It works to relax the intestinal muscles and treat constipation.

In a study , it was found that a mixture of fennel oil with turmeric contributed to the positive treatment of irritable bowel syndrome symptoms. After thirty days, the participants felt that the symptoms had disappeared, they felt less abdominal pain, and they felt more comfortable and their quality of life had improved.

Another study also showed   that mixing fennel with caraway seeds and mint contributed significantly to the treatment of irritable bowel syndrome. It is generally prepared by using two tablespoons of fennel seed powder with a large cup of hot water and leaving them to mix well for ten minutes. Or by using fennel bags.

4. Chamomile tea

Chamomile is one of the herbs for treating irritable bowel syndrome and treating many medical conditions. A study was conducted, the results of which showed that chamomile has strong anti-inflammatory properties, and that it contributes to relaxing the intestinal muscles, treating intestinal disorders, and expelling gases. It is prepared by; Use chamomile bags or fresh or dried leaves to make tea.

5. Turmeric tea

Turmeric is famous for its distinctive therapeutic benefits, especially in treating digestive problems. One study showed that people who took turmeric capsules significantly reduced the symptoms of irritable bowel syndrome, and got rid of abdominal pain and intestinal upset after taking it for 8 weeks. It is usually used by using fresh turmeric or its powder. To make tea, it is a colon herb.

6. Other herbs to treat irritable bowel syndrome

There may be some herbs that make claims about treating colon symptoms, but the evidence for them is still weak, or there is no real scientific evidence about treating colon symptoms. Examples include:

Dandelion tea.

Licorice.

Ginger tea .

Nettle tea.

lavender.

Benefits of drinking herbal tea to treat colon

There are many benefits that drinking various herbs to treat irritable bowel syndrome may bring you, but in general there is a group of them related to colon treatment, which are:

Herbal tea helps relax and reduces psychological stress

It helps relax the intestinal muscles and treat intestinal cramps

Increase the amount of fluid intake, which regulates the functioning of the digestive system .

Being drunk hot contributes to resting the digestive system and facilitating the digestion process

Increase sexual desire with herbs

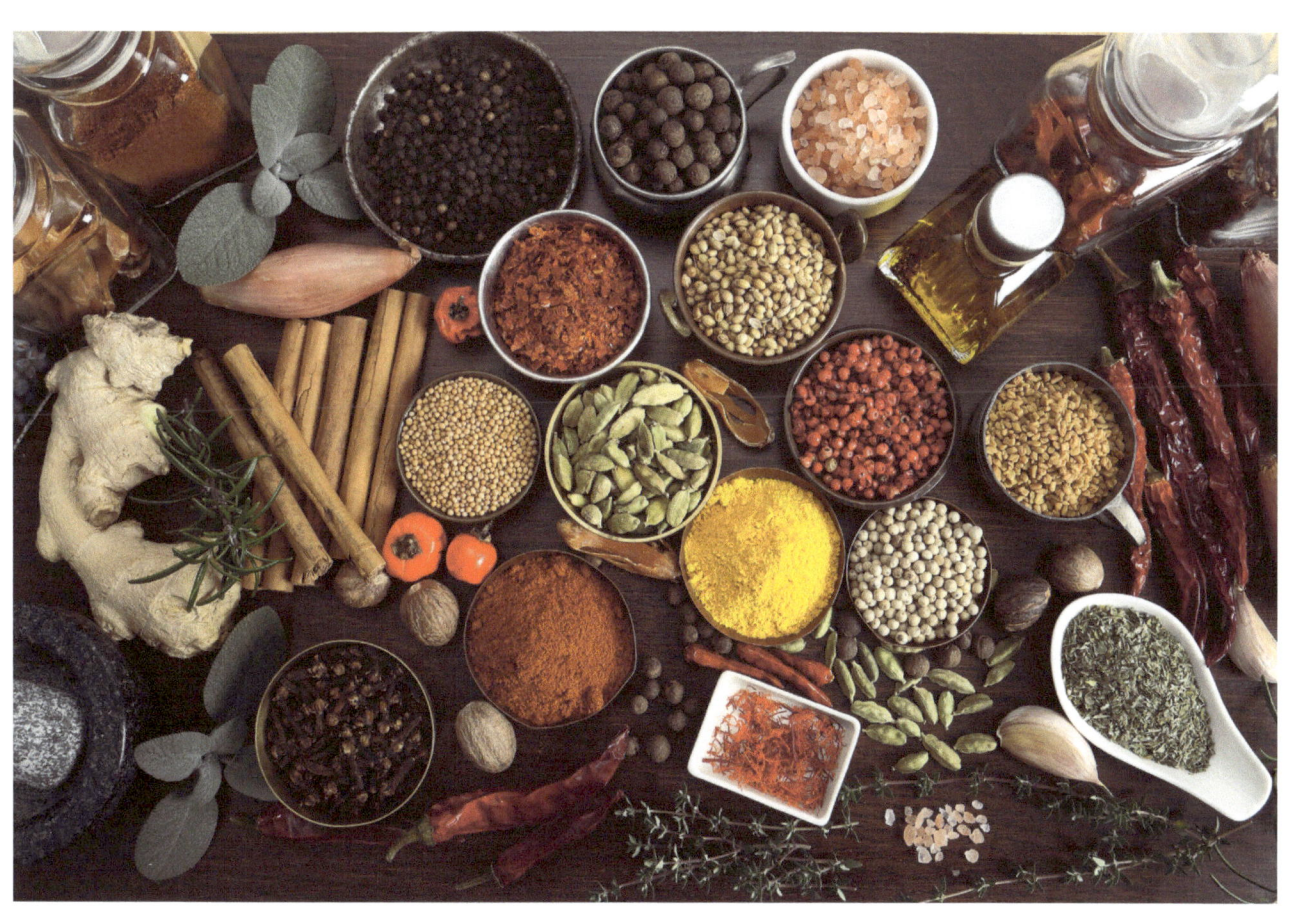

Medicinal herbs may help you increase your sexual desire. Follow the article to learn about ways to increase sexual desire with herbs.

Let us learn in the following about ways to increase sexual desire with herbs and their side effects:

Increase sexual desire with herbs
Often some people suffer from a problem with sexual function or a lack of sexual desire, but is it possible to treat this with medical herbs? Yes, there is a group of herbs that may contribute to increasing sexual desire.

Here are ways to increase sexual desire with herbs :

1. Mandragora officinalis

The Arabs call it "Mandrake apple" and it is a unique and effective plant, and the part that is used for treatment is the fruit of the plant.

In addition to its qualities of stimulating sexual desire and masculine strength, yarrow is also known as a plant that helps relieve pain.

This perennial plant is from the Solanaceae family. It is found on almost all coasts of the Mediterranean Sea. Its root is thick and branched. It resembles the human body and can grow up to two meters in length. The leaves are wide, wrinkled, and have an unpleasant odor.

It has been found that the seeds contain estrogen and are therefore attributed with medicinal properties, and it is known to have the property of arousing love, like Sildenafil these days.

2. Ginseng (Panax)

There are many properties attributed to ginseng roots of all types.

Ginseng root is also known as the "King of Roots", as the age of its roots is very important, and the prevailing belief is that the older it is, the stronger its effect will be.

Ginseng has been known for centuries as having powerful medicinal properties and is used around the world to improve quality of life and health.

There are about 13 different types of ginseng, the most common are:

Korean Asian ginseng (Panax ginseng).
American ginseng (Panax quinquefolium).
Siberian ginseng (Eleuthrococcus senticosus).
Ginseng has a stimulating and strengthening characteristic as it balances the body's systems, and therefore it may:

Helps restore and improve healthy sexual activity.

It stimulates sexual arousal and increases masculine strength.

It affects blood circulation, which is especially important when there are problems with erection .

In addition, ginseng is one of the ways to increase sexual desire with herbs, as it:

Improves the ability of the immune system.

Improves overall feeling and ability to withstand harsh conditions (physical or psychological).

Increase the body's resistance to physical and mental stress (stress).

Reduces irritability, fatigue, weakness and exhaustion.

It affects and strengthens the nervous (psychological/cognitive) system.

It slows down the aging process and improves memory .

Ginseng also has an enhancing and supportive effect on heart function, and it helps and relieves anxiety, stress and depression, factors that often affect sexual function.

3. Herb maca (Lepidium meyenii)

Maca, also known as Peruvian ginseng, is actually a carrot-like, yellow-purple, sweet-tasting edible vegetable used by Indians living above the Andes.

It belongs to the radish family and has amazing active and energetic properties. It grows in the Andes Mountains and is the only one capable of surviving at an altitude of 4000 meters above sea level, hence its enormous health value for the human body.

The Maca plant stimulates, enhances and balances the physical and mental aspects, and is a source of strength and energy. Because it naturally contains vitamins, minerals and essential amino acids. Among its most important benefits:

Helps with hormonal balance for men and women.

Improves focus, cognitive skills, alertness and memory.

Improves fertility in men and women.

It helps in performing physical and sports activity.

It reduces the aging process and improves the quality of life for the elderly.

It increases sexual ability and improves orgasm in both sexes.

When the plant is dried, it will be able to survive for several years without losing its nutritional value, and it contains active substances and most amino acids.

Are methods of increasing libido with herbs always effective?

It cannot be said that the aforementioned herbs are always effective, as they may only contribute to increasing sexual desire in some cases. As for medical cases in which sexual desire is very weak, a doctor should be consulted here.

Are there any harm to ways to increase sexual desire with herbs?

Yes, taking the above herbs in large quantities, without consulting a doctor, may lead to all of the following:

Allergic reaction: Many people suffer from allergies to herbs, and they appear in one of its forms, such as: itching, shortness of breath, skin rash, and the spread of blisters.

Interactions with some medications: The previous herbs may interact with the medication being taken, causing many harms to the body.

Digestive system disorders: Herbs may cause problems in the digestive process, leading to diarrhea or constipation.

Clot-dissolving herbs learn about them

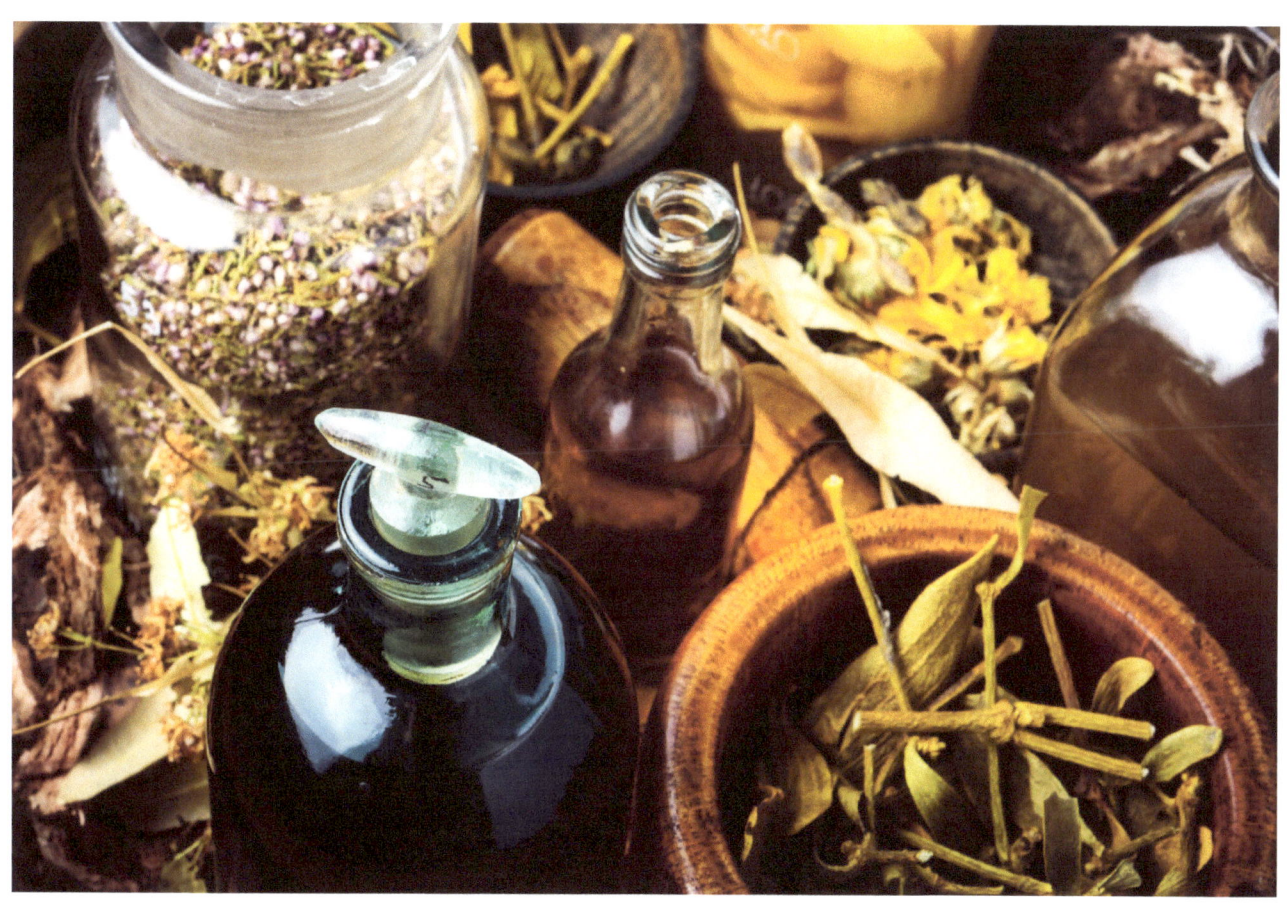

Some people may resort to using herbs that help dissolve clots and protect against thrombosis. Here is the most important information about clot-dissolving herbs in the article.

Blood clotting is a very important process in the body, as it works to stop bleeding and heal wounds, but excessive blood clotting causes many health problems, most notably clots.

Let us learn in the following a list of clot-dissolving herbs in addition to many important information about clots:

Clot-dissolving herbs

There are many anticoagulant medications that some patients who are more at risk of clots need than others, but some people may look for alternative medicine represented by herbs.

Clot-dissolving herbs include the following:

Turmeric

Turmeric may have anticoagulant and anti-inflammatory properties, due to it containing curcumin.

Turmeric can be added to food or drunk with warm water. Both methods will provide benefits.

Cat's claw (Uncaria tomentosa)

One of the clot-dissolving herbs is cat's claw, as cat's claw can help prevent the formation of clots by increasing blood flow in the vessels, and thus may reduce the risk of heart attacks and strokes.

Ginger

Ginger contains salicylate, which helps dissolve clots and prevent clotting.

It is worth noting that aspirin , the common treatment for protection against heart attacks and strokes, was originally manufactured from acetylsalicylic acid, which is derived from salicylates.

Despite this information, there is a need for more research on ways to use and prove the effectiveness of ginger in dissolving clots and preventing clotting.

Red pepper

Red pepper may help dissolve clots and prevent clotting because it also contains high amounts of salicylates, but due to its intense heat, it may not be tolerable for many people.

Red pepper can also help lower blood pressure, increase blood circulation, and relieve pain .

Ginkgo Biloba

Clot-dissolving herbs, one of which is Ginkgo Biloba, as Ginkgo Biloba is one of the herbs used since ancient times to treat blood problems, memory problems, and lethargy.

It has been found that ginkgo can help dissolve clots, but there is still a need to prove this with more studies.

the Garlic

Garlic contains active substances, such as: Ajoene, which may help dissolve clots and prevent clotting. Garlic also has antimicrobial properties.

Cinnamon

Cinnamon contains Coumarin, which is the active ingredient in the widely used drug Warfarin to protect against clots and blood clots.

Cinnamon powder can be added to food, or soak cinnamon sticks in boiling water and drink the infusion.

Chrysanthemum (Chrysanthemum)

One of the clot-dissolving herbs is chrysanthemum, as it may help dissolve clots and prevent clotting by preventing the activity and aggregation of platelets.

Chrysanthemum is an ancient medicinal herb, which has also been used to relieve migraine pain , digestive problems, and high body temperature.

A note about clot-dissolving herbs

Clot-dissolving herbs have become known, but it should be noted that herbs may sometimes help in dissolving clots, but they will not be a substitute for medications due to the lack of sufficient and proven scientific evidence yet.

Also, the use of any of the herbs mentioned above requires medical advice because of its drug interactions that may be dangerous.

Important information about blood clots

Below is a set of important information about blood clots:

Dehydration is one of the causes of clots, so you must drink sufficient amounts of water and other fluids daily.

There are many medications that may lead to the formation of clots, including hormonal medications, such as birth control pills .

Obesity is one of the most prominent causes of clot formation. Clot-dissolving herbs can be used to lose weight, as some of them are effective in this, such as ginger.

Smoking is one of the important causes of clots, especially clots in the lungs.

Treatment of vomiting with herbs

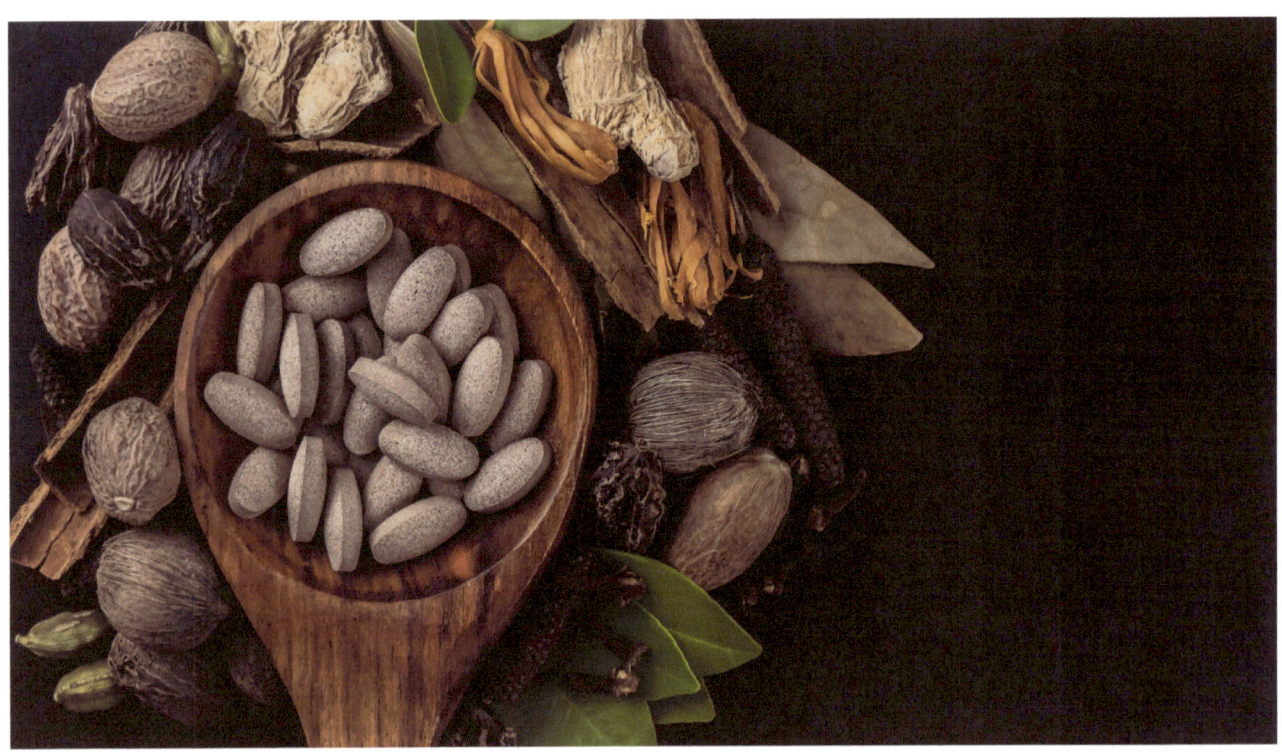

Vomiting is one of the side effects of many digestive system diseases and disorders. Can vomiting be treated with herbs?

Here is the most important information about treating vomiting with herbs:

Treatment of vomiting with herbs
Many people may resort to using herbs to treat their health problems, especially digestive system problems.

There are many studies that show the role of herbs in treating and alleviating nausea and vomiting, but of course, before trying any type of natural herbs, it is necessary to consult a doctor to find out the real cause of nausea and vomiting, and to avoid side effects and drug interactions.

Here are the herbs that may help treat vomiting:

1. Ginger

Ginger is one of the most famous medicinal herbs that helps in treating nausea and vomiting. This is because ginger contains gingerols and shogaols, which affect serotonin and choline receptors, contribute to relaxing the stomach muscles and help expel toxins from the digestive system, thus reducing From vomiting.

2. Peppermint

Peppermint drink also helps reduce nausea and vomiting, due to its properties that help soothe and relax the muscles of the stomach and digestive system. Its aromatic scent also helps relieve symptoms.

A 2013 study indicated a role for peppermint extracts in reducing the severity and frequency of vomiting in cancer patients undergoing chemotherapy .

3. Cinnamon

Cinnamon is one of the herbs that helps relieve and treat digestive disorders. It has soothing properties for the digestive system and stomach muscles. Eating cinnamon contributes to reducing nausea, vomiting, abdominal pain, gas, and indigestion.[

4. Cloves

Eating clove extracts helps relieve nausea, vomiting, and indigestion, due to its stimulating properties of blood circulation and metabolic processes. It also helps in ridding the mouth of bad odor.

5. Cardamom

Taking cardamom extracts helps enhance the health of the digestive system, contributing to reducing stomach acidity, treating nausea, vomiting, indigestion, and abdominal cramps.

6. Asafoetida

Asafoetida herbs help regulate the functioning of the digestive system, and have antiviral and antibacterial properties, thus helping to treat vomiting and diarrhea resulting from infections. You can add asafoetida herbs to warm water or add it with other spices to food.

7. Basil

Basil has anti-colic and anti-spasm properties, helps strengthen the stomach muscles, and contributes to resistance to many diseases that may affect it. Thus reducing vomiting and diarrhea resulting from these diseases.

8. Other herbs to treat vomiting

Here are some other herbs that may help treat vomiting:

Chamomile .
Shumer.
Cumin.
Anise.

How to use herbs

After learning about the ways to treat vomiting with herbs, here are some ways to prepare herbs at home:

Ginger drink

It is prepared as follows:

1-Grate one and a half teaspoons of fresh ginger.

2-Boil 4 cups of water.

3-Add ginger to the boiling water.

4-Remove the water from the heat, then leave the ginger to steep for 5 to 10 minutes.

5-Strain the drink from the ginger pieces, then leave it to cool before drinking it.

Mint drink

He was attended as follows:

1-Boil two cups of water.

2-Add 15 to 20 mint leaves .

3-Turn off the heat, then leave the mint to steep for 10 to 15 minutes.

4-Drink a mint drink with honey and lemon.

Cinnamon drink

Follow these steps:

1-Place a cinnamon stick in a cup.

2-Add boiling water and cover the cup for 10 minutes.

3-Place a tea bag and steep the brew for two minutes as well.

4-Remove the cinnamon stick and tea bag from the drink and add honey if you like.

Clove drink

Follow these steps:

1-Grind a tablespoon of cloves.

2-Boil 4 cups of water.

3-Add boiling water to the ground cloves, and steep for 20 minutes.

4-Strain the drink and it is ready.

Tips on treating vomiting

After learning about the methods of treating vomiting with herbs, here are the most important tips and instructions that will help you relieve vomiting:

Work on stomach comfort

The first step that may help reduce vomiting resulting from inflammation or infection of the digestive system is to try to relax the stomach muscles after vomiting by stopping eating or drinking for 15 to 20 minutes after vomiting.

Eat meals and water gradually

After the stomach is relieved and vomiting does not return, you should start drinking water gradually by drinking a small amount every 5 to 10 minutes. It is preferable to avoid milk and soft drinks at this stage.

Start eating foods approximately 8 to 12 hours after vomiting stops after drinking liquids, and start eating foods that are easy to digest, such as: bananas , rice, apple juice, and toast, and avoid acidic and fatty foods.

Stop medications that irritate the stomach

If you are taking some oral medications that may cause stomach irritation and vomiting again, you must partially stop taking them until the vomiting stops.

Treating delayed pregnancy with herbs

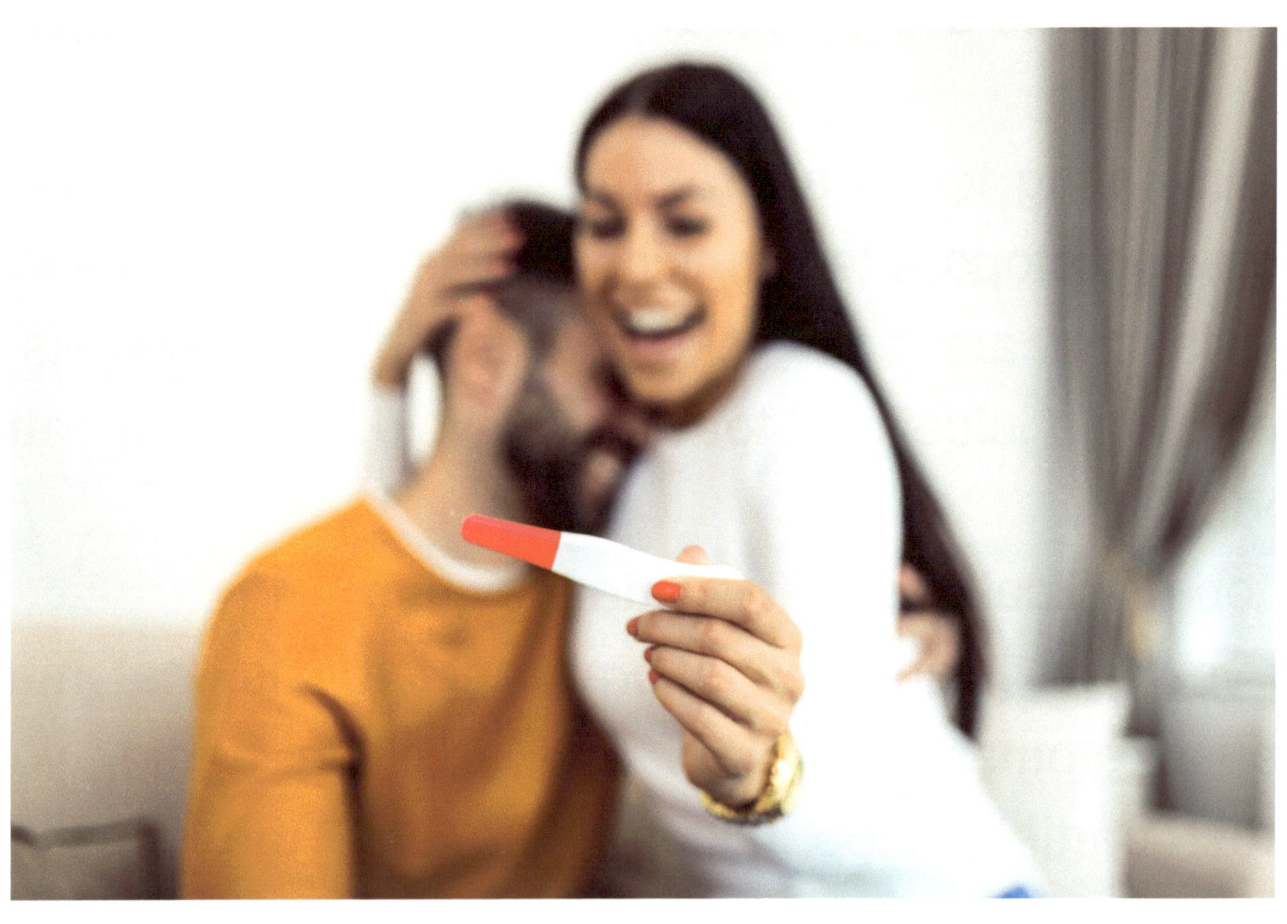

Many women suffer from delayed pregnancy due to many different reasons, but the good news is that it is possible to treat this delay through some medical and natural methods, and in the following article we will discuss treating delayed pregnancy with herbs:

Delayed pregnancy usually occurs as a result of one of the spouses suffering from infertility, which affects the male or female reproductive system, as it is defined by the failure to achieve pregnancy after 12 months or more of regular, unprotected intercourse.

But is it possible to treat delayed pregnancy with herbs?

Treating delayed pregnancy with herbs

Some specialist doctors or health care providers may resort to using some medicinal herbs in order to treat delayed pregnancy and increase the rate of fertility, whether by applying them to women or men. The most prominent examples of treating delayed pregnancy with herbs are the following:

1. Treating delayed pregnancy with herbs for women
Which usually includes the following herbs:

Vitex : The plant may improve female fertility due to its potential effect on prolactin levels. It is often used for women who suffer from a problem in the luteal phase or the second half of the menstrual cycle , according to the results of some studies .

Red clover: According to many fertility experts, it has been found that red clover may help produce follicles and eggs and prepare the body for ovulation, as it is the main ingredient in some types of popular fertility supplements.

Black cohosh: The importance of this type of herb lies in promoting a strong and healthy uterine lining. It helps improve and enhance fertility , in addition to controlling painful periods due to its anti-inflammatory properties.

Siberian ginseng: It is a relatively good herb in the field of fertility, as it is known for its ability to fight fatigue and normalize hormonal balance in females. Which contributes to enhancing fertility.

2. Treating delayed pregnancy with herbs for men

It is possible that the reason behind delayed pregnancy is the presence of a problem in men. Here are the most prominent herbs for treating delayed pregnancy in men:

Ashwagandha: Many studies have shown that this herb helps enhance male fertility and sperm health, as it works to increase sperm count and motility, in addition to increasing levels of reproductive hormones.

Fenugreek: Fenugreek extract was found to have clearly helped increase testosterone levels, improving the shape and production of sperm at the same time.

Shilajit: This herb may improve infertility and increase male hormone levels .

Treating delayed pregnancy naturally

After discussing the most prominent methods used to treat delayed pregnancy with herbs, here are the following are the most prominent methods used to treat delayed pregnancy that some may suffer from naturally:

Eating foods that contain antioxidants, for example: folic acid and zinc, is sufficient to improve fertility in both men and women.

Eat a large breakfast, especially for women who suffer from some fertility problems.

Eating healthy fats daily may help enhance fertility, and it is also important to know that trans fats may sometimes increase the risk of ovulatory infertility.

Reduce the intake of foods that contain carbohydrates, especially if the woman suffers from polycystic ovary syndrome (PCOS).

Eat plenty of fiber, as it helps the body get rid of excess hormones, in addition to maintaining blood sugar balance.

Replacing animal proteins with plant proteins may play a role in reducing the risk of infertility.

Treating premature ejaculation with herbs and natural methods

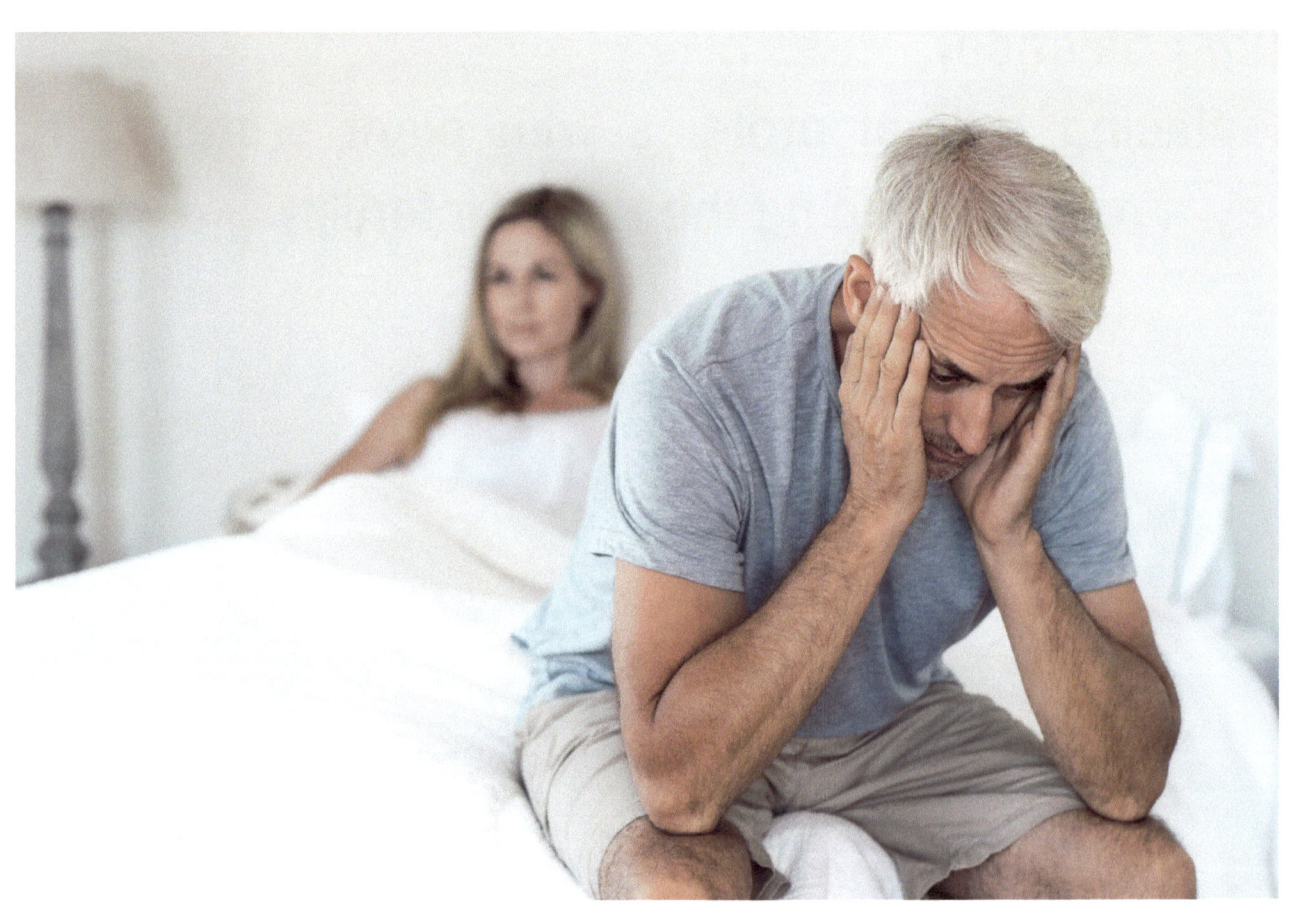

Premature ejaculation is a very common condition in men, as it may return to childbirth and sometimes develop with age. We have brought to you the most important methods of treating premature ejaculation with herbs.

Premature ejaculation is a condition in which a man reaches his climax before he or his partner wants to. It is a very common condition in males, so we have brought to you, dear man, the best ways to treat premature ejaculation with herbs.

Treating premature ejaculation with herbs

There are various herbs that increase the time you need to reach orgasm:

1. Asparagus

The benefits of the asparagus plant are varied , including its importance for heart health and its ability to act as an anti-depressant. However, the most important thing that asparagus is famous for is its effectiveness in promoting sexual health.

You can consume asparagus either alone or within various meals, while its benefits are beneficial to the sexual health of men and women, and are not limited to men only.

2. Hibiscus

Hibiscus is a very popular drink in some Arab countries. Its color tends to be pink, and it contains a high percentage of vitamin C. Because hibiscus contains vitamin C, it greatly enhances sexual health, as it improves erection and slows down the ejaculation process. Therefore, it is very useful in treating premature ejaculation with herbs.

3. Ginseng

The ginseng plant is famous for its effectiveness for men and women, as it enhances sexual desire in women and strengthens erection in men. Also, using it in a cream and placing it on the penis an hour before intercourse slows down premature ejaculation.

4. Treating premature ejaculation with Ayurvedic herbal medicine

Ayurveda is a system of Indian folk medicine, dating back thousands of years, that uses specific herbs to treat every disease.

It is believed that Ayurvedic herbs are able to treat premature ejaculation if they are used twice daily, in the form of a capsule in lukewarm water, and in ancient Indian medicine it was used to treat erectile dysfunction.

One study conducted in 2017 and published in the online scientific journal Science Direct found that these herbs actually have a slight, but important, effect in increasing the time it takes a man to ejaculate. Therefore, it helps in treating premature ejaculation with herbs.

5. Treating premature ejaculation with Chinese herbs
Imzosec tablets, or Qilin pills in particular, among other Chinese herbal medicines, take them daily or even weekly to treat premature ejaculation, by enhancing sexual stamina.

The same study mentioned previously found that Chinese herbal medicines can increase the time it takes a man to ejaculate by about two minutes.

6. Zinc supplements
Zinc from nutrition enhances immunity and cell growth, in addition, it helps produce testosterone and enhance libido.

Some research has found a link between zinc deficiency and sexual dysfunction in men, as taking 11 milligrams of zinc daily may improve the time of ejaculation and help treat premature ejaculation with herbs.

7. Nutrition

In addition to zinc in nutrition, magnesium also plays a role in enhancing your sexual health and in controlling premature ejaculation. According to research, consuming foods rich in zinc and magnesium may help with the same goal.

Among these foods you will find:

Oysters.
Pumpkin.
Soybeans .
Spinach.
Loose.
Beans.
the Garlic.
Dark chocolate.
Other steps have proven effective
Here are some other simple steps proven to help treat premature ejaculation with herbs:

1. Topical anesthetic creams and sprays

These creams and sprays do not require a prescription, and they contain a local anesthetic agent that, when applied to the penis, reduces the intensity of sensation. Thus reducing the speed of reaching orgasm.

Usually, the cream is applied to the penis 10–15 minutes before intercourse, as this is enough to add a few minutes to the time of ejaculation.

2. Temporary compression technique

It is very possible that the technique of temporary pressure on the penis will serve you to delay the ejaculation process.

When you feel unwanted ejaculation approaching, ask your partner to press the end of the penis, where the head joins the shaft, for several seconds until you feel a decrease in climax.

You can repeat this process until you find that the time is right for ejaculation and then delay it until the time you prefer, as this helps in treating premature ejaculation with herbs.

3. Interruption and continuity technique

Another way to control your sexual climax is to completely stop intercourse when you reach climax, which interrupts the pleasure. When you feel that you have become less aroused, you can resume intercourse.

Of course, stopping this does not mean that you will cut off from your wife completely, but rather you can invest this time in caressing her and inciting her sense of pleasure.

4. Pelvic floor exercises

Kegel exercises or pelvic floor exercises help strengthen your pelvic floor muscles, making you able to control them better. Thus controlling how much you feel during intercourse.

It has been shown that pelvic floor exercises can help men who suffer from premature ejaculation control it better. Therefore, it helps in treating premature ejaculation with herbs.

5. Condoms

Condoms in general reduce the feeling of arousal as they form a buffer between the penis and foreplay and friction. However, in addition to the usual condoms, you can find a special condom made to treat premature ejaculation. Go to the pharmacy near you and inquire about it from the pharmacist.

Herbs that help sleep a list of the most important ones

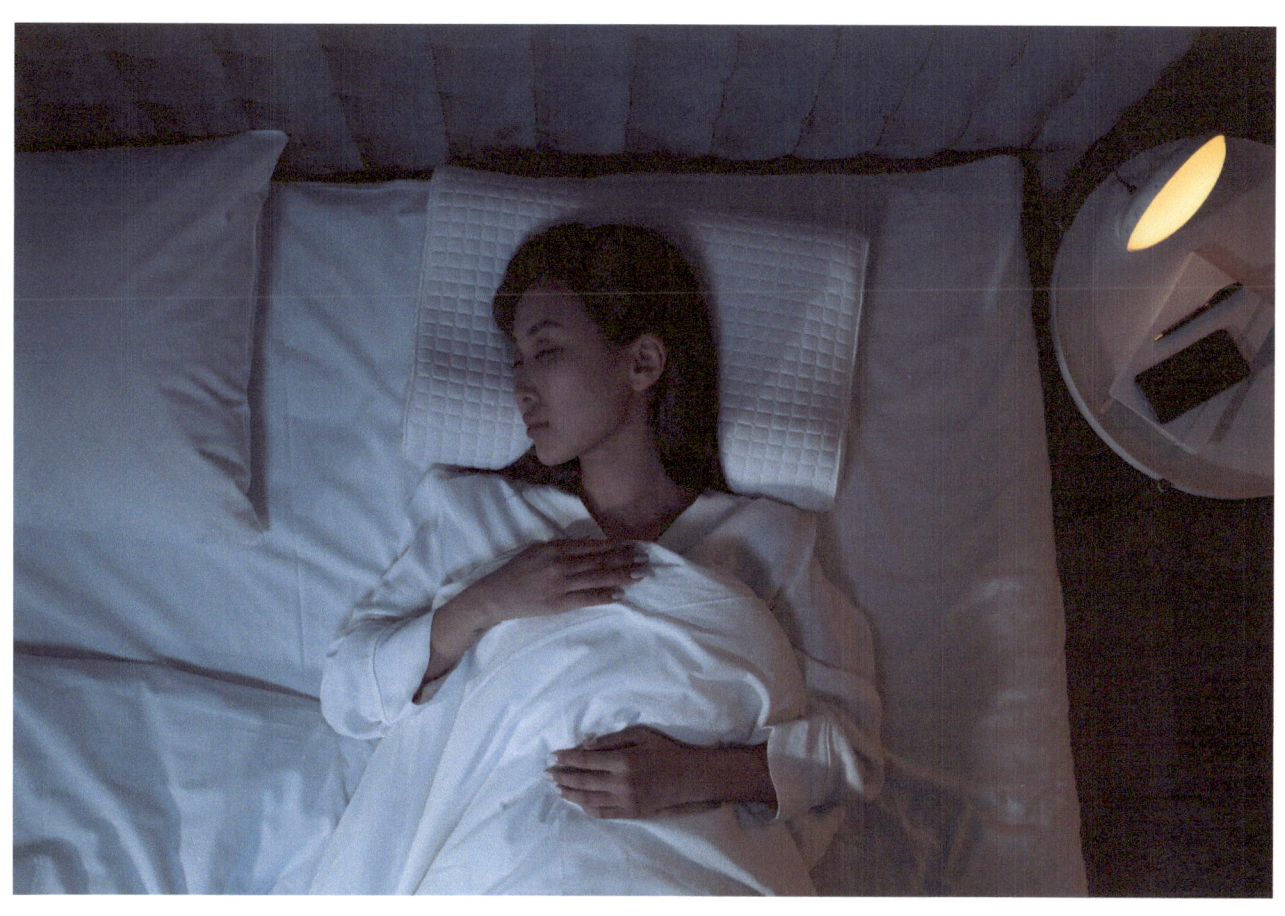

Do you suffer from insomnia and an inability to sleep as deeply as you should? In this article, we will review a list of herbs that help sleep.

Getting an adequate amount of sleep at night every day is very important because sleep has many benefits . Here we will enumerate for you a group of herbs that help you sleep:

Herbs that help you sleep

There are many plants and herbs that eating or drinking their infusion will help you get a good night's sleep, the most important of which are:

1. Chamomile

It is preferable to take a decoction of chamomile before bed to get a good night's sleep. One study has proven that chamomile actually helps with sleep.

One study also showed that mothers taking chamomile decoction regularly before bedtime greatly helped them sleep, relieve symptoms of depression , and relax.

2. Violet flower

Violets are a plant with beautiful violet flowers characterized by their wonderful scent and many health and beauty benefits. You do not have to eat violets to obtain their sleep benefits, as simply inhaling the scent of violet essential oil for 30 minutes before bed effectively helps with sleep, improves its quality, and gets rid of insomnia.

3. Valerian root

Valerian root, also known as valerian, is one of the medicinal plants with many therapeutic benefits. It has a wonderful anesthetic and sedative effect, which makes it included in our list of herbs that help with sleep.

It is possible to benefit from valerian either by taking special supplements containing the extract of this plant, or by drinking a decoction of this plant.

A decoction of valerian is often combined with a decoction of chamomile, which is a mixture that helps calm the nerves and nerve cells in the brain , which reduces insomnia and helps sleep.

4. John's Wort

Since depression is one of the causes of insomnia and the inability to sleep properly, the saintly herb greatly helps with sleep because of its ability to improve mood and prevent depression.

The relationship between insomnia and depression is strong, and each may lead to the other, so using saintly herb is very useful for combating both.

5. Lemon balm plant

Lemon balm is a member of the mint family . It is a common plant spread around the world, and its leaves can be used both dried and fresh.

One study has found that the lemon balm plant actually has a narcotic effect, and it is one of the herbs that helps sleep and relieve insomnia if a few sips of a decoction of the leaves are taken regularly before bed.

6. Red passion flower (Passiflora incarnata)

A passion flower decoction is made using the dried leaves of this flower or the petals of the flower itself. The red passion flower has been used since ancient times to treat insomnia and improve sleep.

Sometimes doctors resort to using a mixture of valerian and passion flower as an ideal medicine to improve sleep quality when drinking the decoction regularly for at least a week.

7. Bark of magnolia

The magnolia plant is one of the very ancient plants that humans have known since ancient times for its benefits that help with sleep. Magnolia bark was also commonly used in ancient Chinese civilization for several health purposes, such as: abdominal pain and nasal congestion .

You can benefit from the benefits of magnolia bark for sleep by drinking a decoction of the bark regularly.

8. Other herbs that help sleep

There are also a group of herbs, substances, spices, and even fruits that may help you sleep as well, such as: turmeric, ginger, cinnamon, and mint.

These are some herbal recipes that help with sleep:

Boil a banana with its peel for 10 minutes, then drink the resulting water before bedtime regularly.

Boil a little turmeric with a handful of cloves and cinnamon, and add a little honey to the mixture.

Place three cloves of garlic in the water. As soon as the water starts to boil, turn off the heat and add a little honey and lemon juice to the warm water.

When should you be careful?

After learning about herbs that help sleep, it is important to note the importance of always paying attention to the following things before starting to take any of the herbs mentioned above:

Start by eating very small amounts to ensure that you do not suffer from any type of allergy to these herbs.

Stop taking these herbs immediately if you notice any side effects.

Consult your doctor about any herbs you intend to take with this medication for fear of any complications arising if you are taking medication prescribed by your doctor for sleep.

Treating insomnia with medicinal herbs a list of the most important ones

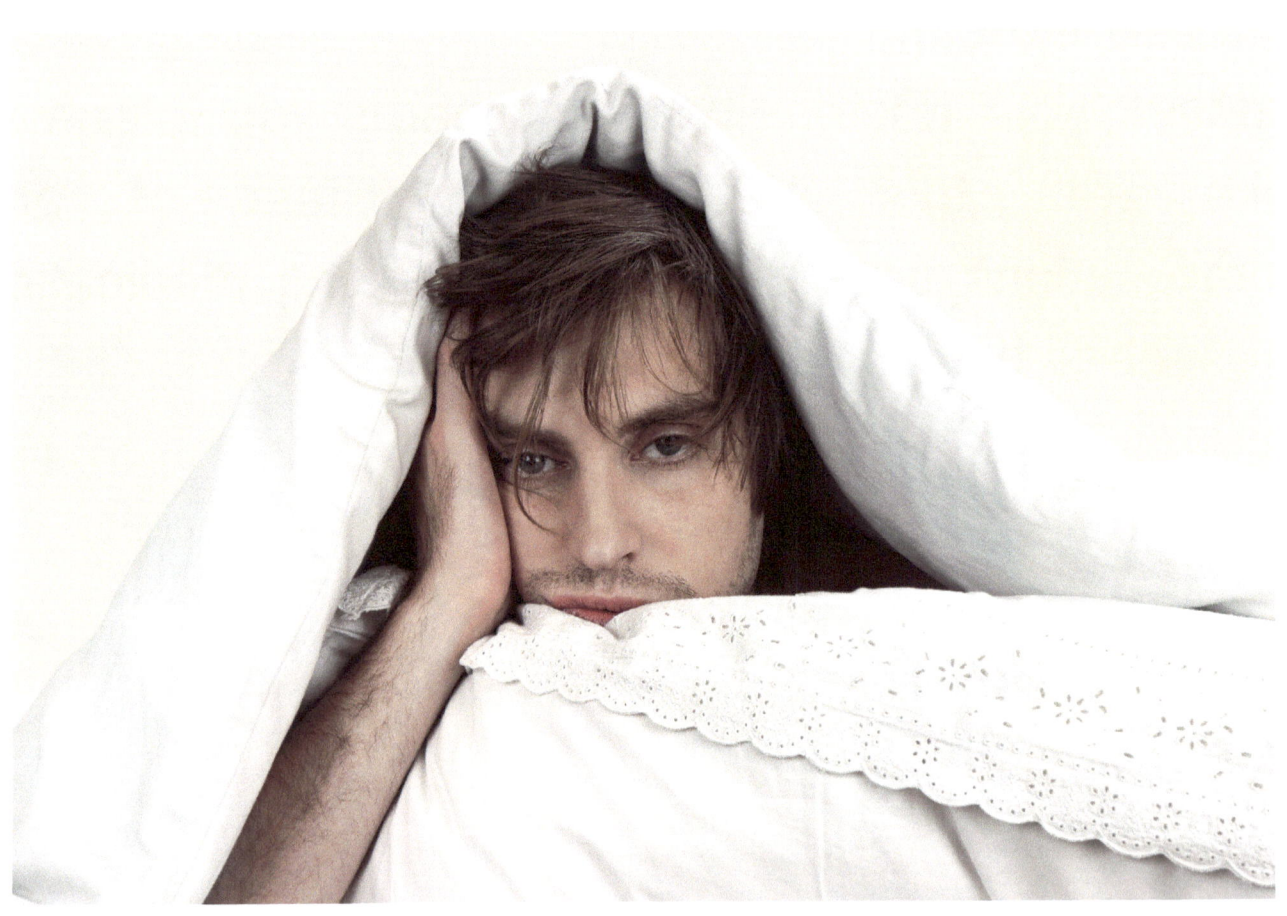

Chronic insomnia may greatly disrupt our lives, but insomnia can be treated with medicinal herbs that enable you to get uninterrupted sleep throughout the night. Here are the most important of these herbs.

Insomnia often comes in two forms: either the person finds it difficult to sleep and tries to sleep but remains completely awake, or insomnia occurs in the hours after midnight.

Many people suffer from insomnia due to a stressful lifestyle, improper diet, and artificial lighting from computer screens and smartphones. Many people resort to taking sleeping pills to get rid of insomnia, but can insomnia be treated with herbs?

Treating insomnia with herbs

Insomnia can be treated with medical herbs in its various cases, whether it is difficulty sleeping or waking up spontaneously in the middle of the night. There are a group of herbs available that help get rid of insomnia and improve sleep quality. We mention some of them as follows:

1. Valerian (Valeriana officinalis)

Valerian, or what is known as valerian, is recommended for calm and relaxation , and it also helps in getting a better quality of sleep and falling asleep faster.

However, you must consult a specialist doctor regarding the recommended dose of valerian. Because it may interact with some medications, in addition to being unsafe for pregnant women and children.

2. California poppy (Eschscholzia californica)

California poppy is one of the options for treating insomnia with herbs. This herb is effective for treating sleep problems, anxiety , various aches, nervous agitations, and many other conditions.

There are not enough studies to prove that California poppy is safe, so check with your doctor before taking it.

3. Red passionflower (Passiflora incarnata)

It is a medicinal herb that is recommended for people who tend to wake up several times during the night, as it helps in the process of regulating sleep and relaxation as well.

It is also used to soothe stomach disorders.

4. Common hops (Humulus lupulus)

Or what is known as hops, is an herb that stimulates sleep and is also effective in treating anxiety and digestive system problems .

This herb is probably safe to use as part of herbal treatment for insomnia, but due to the natural steroids it contains, it is not recommended for pregnant women and children.

5. Chamomile (Matricaria chamomilla)

It is one of the ancient and common medicinal herbs used to treat insomnia and sleep disorders, as chamomile tea is particularly popular and known for its soothing properties.

Chamomile can also be used safely to treat children and adults alike.

The effect of herbs on those who take sleeping pills
If you take sleeping pills regularly, you may discover that these medicinal herbs do not affect you immediately, as your body has become more accustomed to the chemical components found in the sleeping pills.

If you stop taking sleeping pills, their effect will decline, and the body will take a long time to completely eliminate the effect of the drugs, and treating insomnia with medicinal herbs will begin to affect your sleep quality.

Important tips for treating insomnia

Treating insomnia with medicinal herbs can help solve the problem, but in addition to that, it is preferable to adopt some habits that help the body relax and prepare for sleep, including the following:

Eat a light dinner three hours before bed.

Take a shower with warm water 90 minutes before bed. You can use lavender essential oil, as it is recommended during bathing to soothe the body and soul.

Make sure to turn off all lights and screens in the room before sleeping .

Set aside time before bed for silence and meditation.

Try relaxing activities before bed, such as reading a book, having a quiet conversation, or drinking herbal tea.

If you are anxious, write down on a piece of paper everything that is bothering you ; Because recording these thoughts on paper can wonderfully contribute to your psychological calm.

Make sure to get a good, deep sleep at night so that you wake up refreshed and full of energy in the morning.

Treating asthma with herbsproven effective in some cases!

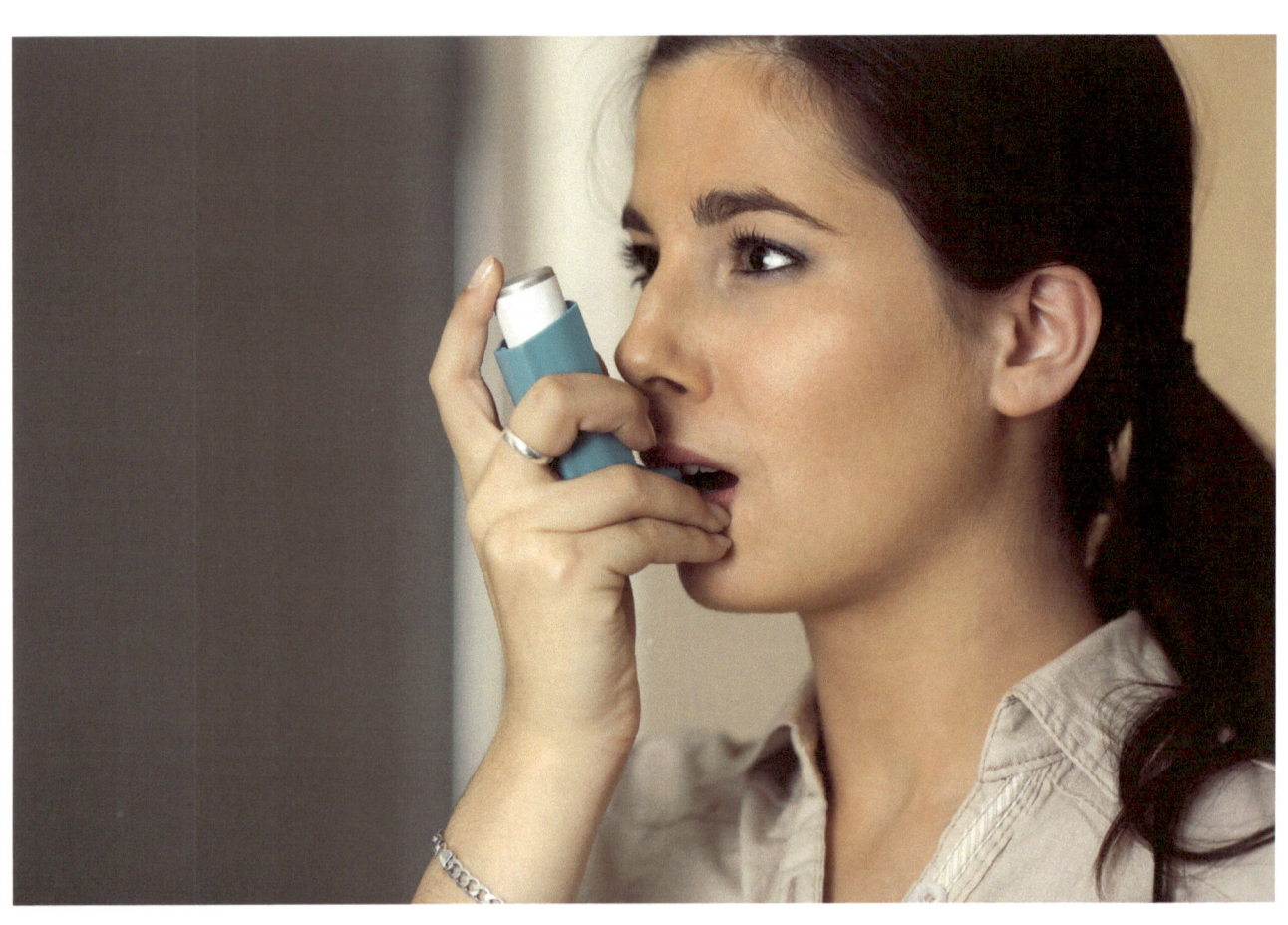

Respiratory infections are one of the most common diseases among preschool children and can be dangerous for adults. Treating asthma with medicinal herbs has proven effective in some cases.

Respiratory pathogens such as asthma, like other diseases, are related to the balance between the ability of germs or viruses to penetrate the body and cause disease, and the body's ability to prevent the entry of germs and stop the development of the disease.

The immune system is made up of different cells with diverse functions. Such as white blood cells that learn to recognize different viruses and produce special antibodies to them.

Therefore, when there is repeated contact between the same viruses, the immune system produces effective antibodies, and thus the disease can disappear easily. Children who have not yet been exposed to various viruses, such as children who have just started attending nursery, have a greater risk of severe infection.

Common symptoms of respiratory tract infection are high fever, cough, sore throat, colds, and more. Children and adults with asthma – an allergic inflammatory condition of the airways – can develop airway inflammation more easily, and in addition, airway inflammation may appear more difficult to develop.

Although antibiotics can help fight bacteria, they are unable to do so against viral infections, which are more common than respiratory tract infections. Here, medicinal herbs enter the picture, including treating asthma with herbs .

Treating asthma with herbs:

One of the advantages of herbal medicine is that it strengthens the immune system. Medicinal herbs improve the condition of the mucous membrane of the respiratory tract and increase the amount of white blood cells. There are also medicinal herbs that work against allergies and help relieve allergic phlegm and spasms in the respiratory tract.

One of the ways to treat asthma with herbs is to use garden iris (Nigella Sativa). This plant is very well known in Asia and is widespread in the Mediterranean. In a traditional way, the seeds of this plant were used to prevent and treat allergic diseases such as asthma.

The substance extracted from the iris plant is taken by drinking, and it prevents attacks of shortness of breath in most people with asthma. The extract is given to children and adults with good results.

Other research has shown the plant's positive effect on other diseases such as colds, eczema, and more. In a study from 2008 conducted on 29 asthma patients, the patients were divided into experimental groups, in which the patients were given the plant extract, and a control group who did not receive the extract. For three months, the researchers examined the groups' asthma severity.

The frequency of attacks, duration of wheezing, respiratory function, which included respiratory airflow speed, lung volume, and more, were measured.
Tests were performed after a month and a half of tracking only, without treatment. After that, the patients received black seed treatment for a month and a half and were examined again.

The condition of the people in the groups improved after treatment with the plant. Inhalation of Ventolin and other substances – decreased significantly over time.

Control groups that did not receive the plant extract had almost no improvement.

In another study conducted in 2009, 84 children with asthma, ages 5–7, who suffered from respiratory tract infections, were examined. Different parameters were examined before and after treatment with the medicinal plant.

The results showed an increase in the ability to breathe, a decrease in the number of breaths per minute, a decrease in the amount of wheezing when breathing, a decrease in respiratory tract obstruction, etc.

Accordingly, various medicinal plants, such as the Nigella sativa plant, have proven their ability to treat asthma with herbs and to prevent and treat respiratory tract infections and cases of asthma effectively and without side effects.

*The plant has additional important treatment capabilities that are not related to inflammation of the respiratory tract.

This article is intended to provide information and does not constitute a prescription for medical treatment.

Strengthening immunity with herbsHere is a group of effective herbs

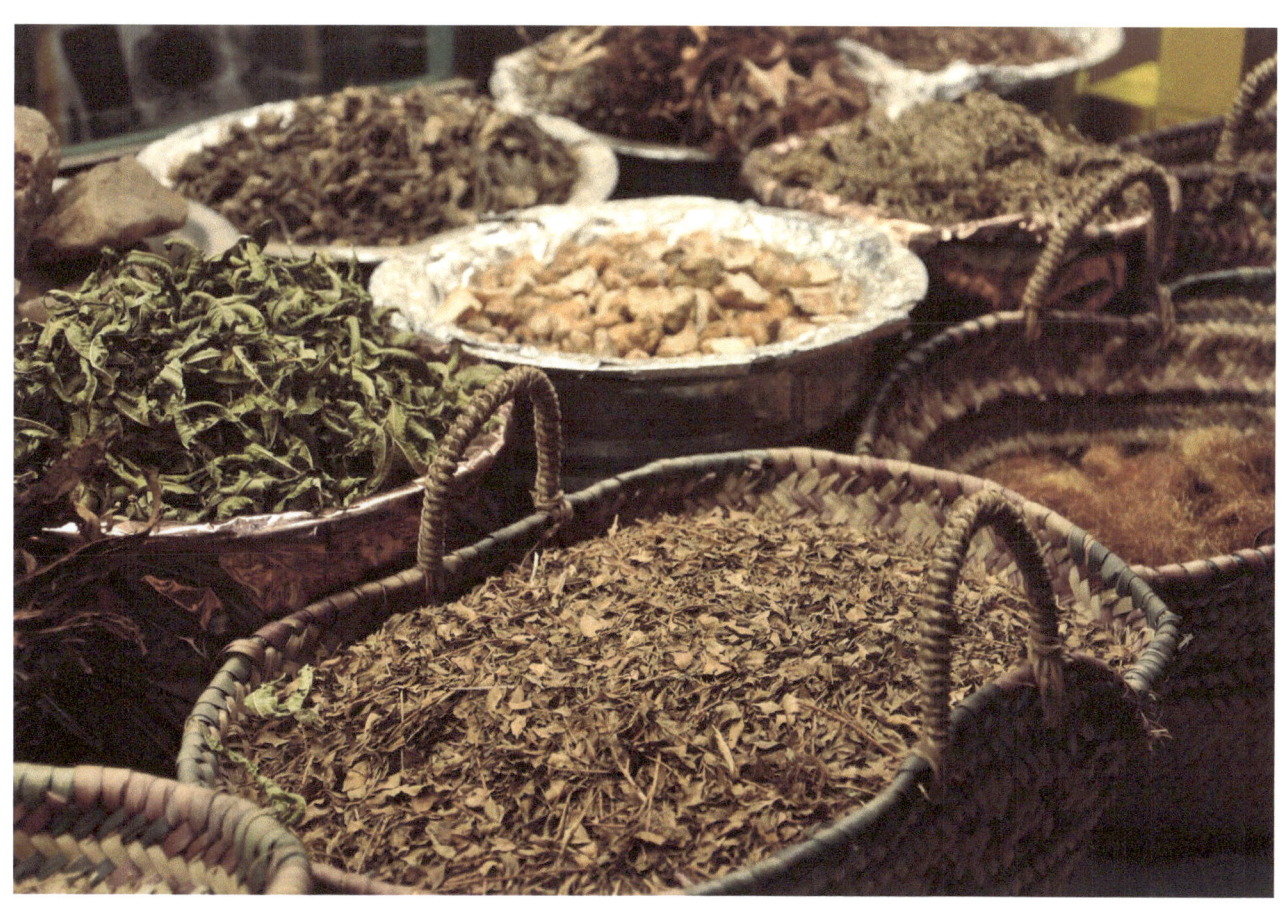

How to strengthen immunity with herbs? What herbs should we eat? What is the correct use of these herbs? You can find all the answers in the article.

Let us learn in the following about ways to strengthen immunity with herbs, in addition to learning how to use these herbs correctly:

Strengthen immunity with herbs

Immunity can be strengthened with the following herbs:

1. Echinacea

The echinacea plant has many types, but purple echinacea (Echinacea purpurea) is considered the most effective among them. It has been found that treatment with this herb reduces the rate of suffering in the upper respiratory tract by 58% and reduces the length of the illness by a day and a half.

This plant is directed to strengthening the immune system. The echinacea plant contains many active substances that affect and activate the immune system, including: substances that may contribute to sterilizing and eliminating viruses and germs.

2. Siberian ginseng (Eleutherococcus senticosus)

Siberian ginseng has wonderful properties and has an effect on most of the body's systems. Much research has been conducted on this plant in the past, and it has been shown that it is particularly effective in preventing diseases that affect the upper respiratory system and influenza.

There is a variety in the quality of Siberian ginseng preparations available in the market, so it is best to know the main source and verify the effectiveness of the product.

Care must be taken to take the preparation at the correct time, as some preparations are recommended to be taken close to mealtime, but taking another preparation at this time may harm the body's absorption of it, so you must carefully read the instructions written on the product to know the appropriate time.

3. Garlic (Allium sativum)

One of the ways to strengthen immunity with herbs is to eat garlic. The use of garlic has been known since the time of the ancient Egyptians, and it has been used in various civilizations around the world to prevent influenza and upper respiratory tract diseases.

Among all the pharmacological effects of garlic, its antibacterial, antiviral, antifungal, and antiparasitic activities are also known.

Many experiments have proven that garlic has more antimicrobial activity than any other antibacterial substance. In addition, its effect enhances the immune system. In one of the studies conducted to determine its therapeutic qualities, it was found that the rate of health disorders among people who ate garlic was lower than others.

4. Social Microtus)

Although propolis is a waxy substance taken from the bee hive, it is considered a medicinal herb

In one of the studies conducted on the use of a mixture of echinacea, propolis and vitamin C, it showed a significant decrease according to statistical standards in the incidence of upper respiratory tract diseases in children.

Correct use of medicinal herbs

The use of medicinal herbs to prevent and treat influenza and respiratory tract infections has been known in the folk medicine of different peoples. Some of these medicinal herbs have been studied, and it has been found that they are indeed effective in shortening the days of illness with influenza or respiratory tract infections.

But it must be noted here that the medicinal herbs on which research was conducted were used in the research conditions in specific ways, in terms of:

Method of administration.
the focus.
Level of quality control.

Therefore, there is great importance in choosing the correct plant and using its parts correctly. It is also important to choose the preparation made from this plant and how to take it according to the instructions attached to the herb or according to the herbal expert.

Many of the herbs that have been studied are available on the market today, but in different concentrations and with different production quality than those under research conditions, so it is possible that the results of using these preparations available on the market will be different from those on which the research was conducted.

It is worth noting that if you follow methods to strengthen immunity with herbs, the body may cause some side effects, including:

Allergic reaction: which appears in several forms, such as: fever, nausea , and skin rash.

Drug interactions: Taking herbs with a medication can be a direct cause of a health condition relapse, which is why it is always recommended to consult a doctor in this regard.

Learn how to treat diarrhea with herbs

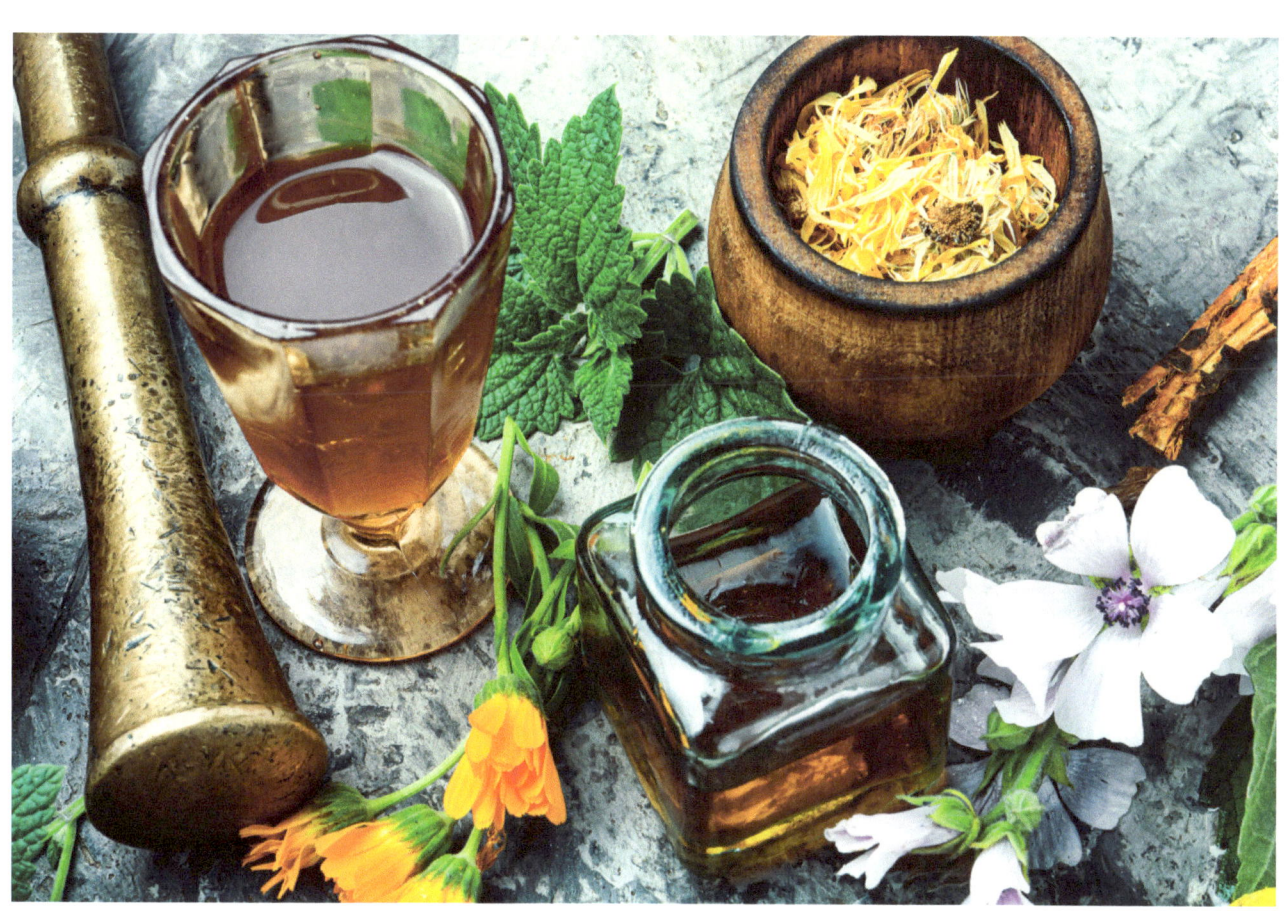

Diarrhea is a common digestive disorder, especially in patients with irritable bowel syndrome. Some people may resort to treating the problem using herbs. Can diarrhea be treated with herbs?

Here is the most important information about treating diarrhea with herbs:

Treating diarrhea with herbs
Some herbs have antidiarrheal properties that may help relieve and reduce diarrhea. However, it must be noted that before consuming any medicinal plants and herbs, it is necessary to consult a doctor in order to reduce side effects and drug interactions.

Here is the most important information about herbs that may help treat and relieve diarrhea:

Chamomile

Chamomile is one of the famous herbs used to treat many diseases and health problems. Drinking chamomile tea or therapeutic capsules may help relieve diarrhea symptoms, relieve digestive system infections, and reduce abdominal cramps and pain.

Berry Leaf

Drinking raspberry leaf tea, whether black, blue, or red raspberry leaves, may also help reduce digestive system inflammation and intestinal secretions, thus alleviating the severity and symptoms of diarrhea.

The reason for this is because mulberry leaves contain tannins, which contribute to this.

Wild mallow (Malva sylvestris)

The flowers and leaves of wild hibiscus are rich in medicinal substances and components, so wild hibiscus helps in reducing diarrhea due to its laxative properties due to it containing astringent tannins.

Wild mallow extracts may help treat: infections, coughs, colds, sore throats, stomach ulcers, constipation, urinary retention, cystitis, and obesity as well.

Mint

Peppermint drink is one of the most useful and popular medicinal drinks. Peppermint oil is used to reduce abdominal cramps and relax the intestines, thus helping to regulate the work of the digestive system and relieving diarrhea.

Cress

Taking garden cress extracts may help treat abdominal disorders resulting from diarrhea and dysentery .

Evidence has indicated that it has anti-diarrheal properties in laboratory animals by activating potassium channels and inhibiting the action of some enzymes within the intestine.

Basil
Basil is also one of the famous herbs, as it helps in treating diarrhea because it contains several substances, such as: saponins, and tannins that help reduce diarrhea.

Other herbs may help treat diarrhea
Here are some other herbs and plants that may help treat diarrhea:

1-Thyme .
2-Turmeric.
Ways to use herbs to treat diarrhea
Here are some ways to prepare homemade herbs to treat diarrhea:

Prepare chamomile drink

Here are the preparation steps:

1-Collect chamomile flowers , wash them with warm water and allow them to dry.

2-Boil a cup of water.

3-Add chamomile flowers to boiling water and steep for 5 minutes.

4-Remove the flowers and pour the syrup into the cup.

Prepare mint drink

Here are the preparation steps:

1-Boil two cups of water.

2-Add approximately 15 mint leaves to the boiling water.

3-Steep the drink 3 to 5 minutes.

4-Add honey if you like.

Preparing red raspberry leaf drink

Preparation steps:

1-Wash two handfuls of raspberries and leaves well.

2-Boil two cups of water.

3-Add raspberry leaves and boil with water for one to two minutes.

4-Soak the mixture for 10 to 15 minutes.

5-Add the berries to the cup and pour the drink.

Home remedies for diarrhea

After you learned about the ways to treat diarrhea with herbs, here are the most important tips and instructions on treating diarrhea at home:

1. Drink plenty of fluids

In the event of severe diarrhea, drinking water helps replace the body with lost fluids and salts, such as sodium.

You can add two teaspoons of salt and 12 teaspoons of sugar to two liters of water, as this helps enhance the health and ability of the intestines to absorb fluids and reduce the risk of dehydration.

2. Take probiotics

Probiotics are nutritional supplements of bacteria that are beneficial to the health and functioning of the digestive system. Eating it can help relieve the severity and symptoms of diarrhea.

But of course, consulting a doctor or pharmacist is necessary.

3. Diet modification

Try to eat small, scattered meals instead of eating a large, fatty meal. It is also preferable to add some foods and avoid others, so that meals should be based on foods that are low in fiber and rich in starches.

Foods that are preferable to eat to treat diarrhea:

Fruits, such as: bananas and apples.
the soup.
Cooked vegetables, such as potatoes.
the rice.
Toast bread.

Foods and drinks to avoid:

Fatty foods rich in fat.

Spicy foods.

Foods full of processed sugars .

Foods full of fructose.

Alarm clocks.

Alcohol.

Soft drinks.

4. Taking medications

There are some pharmaceutical treatments that can be taken without a prescription, such as Loperamide, which helps relieve the severity of diarrhea and speed up treatment.

However, it should not be used before medical or pharmaceutical advice, especially in the case of bloody diarrhea or high temperature.

Herbs for weight loss what are they and how do they work?

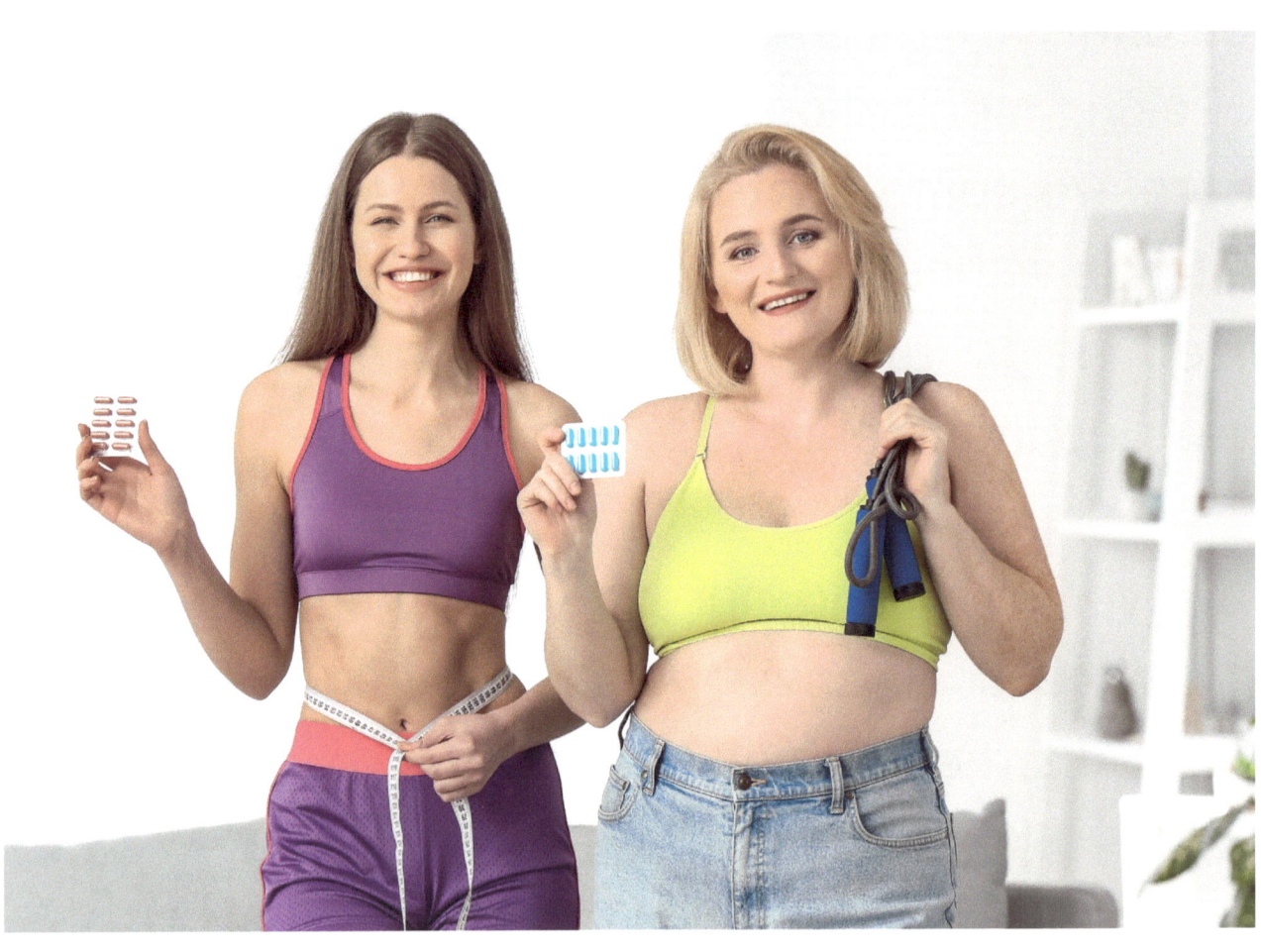

Are you overweight? Do you want to know the most prominent herbs for weight loss that will help you lose weight? So follow the article, to tell you about these herbs and their side effects.

With increased awareness and knowledge, we have become more aware of the best approach that must be followed to lose weight and get rid of obesity , and we must introduce some types of herbs to get rid of excess weight in addition to the diet followed.

Herbs for weight loss and weight loss

From following a healthy lifestyle and gradually losing weight through exercise and an appropriate diet, and most importantly of all, be patient to see the results.

However, unfortunately, many people, despite being aware of the harmful effects of other methods on their health, still have little patience and their need to see quick results, make them rush things and research and try other and new methods, such as:

Hard and fast diet.

Resorting to slimming pills and medications.

Performing surgeries.

Of course, they realize the truth later after facing the harms resulting from misuse, the least of which are:

Depression.

paleness.

Exhaustion.

weakness.

Pressure drop.

Return to twice the weight later.

One of the methods that have become popular and used and are attached to a specific dietary pattern or diet is herbs for weight loss , which science has proven and confirmed to be positive in losing weight, and has classified the side effects resulting from their use, and how this is done.

Below we list some of these herbs that may have an effect on metabolism and appetite:

Cinnamon.
Ginger.
Green tea.
Flax seeds.
Ginseng.

Cinnamon for weight loss

One of the positive things that makes cinnamon one of the herbs for weight loss is that it:

It prevents infections and is anti-fungal and anti-parasitic.

It is an excellent source of dietary fiber , iron , and calcium.

It is successful in lowering blood sugar levels. One of the benefits of cinnamon has been found to be that it slows down the speed of digestion and absorption of food in the intestines, which may reduce high blood sugar levels.

It adds a sweet flavor to foods, which can help discourage cravings for foods, especially sweet ones.

It helps transport fats from the liver, so that the body can use them to obtain energy, and increases the rate of fat metabolism and burns them more easily.

Reducing bad cholesterol (LDL).

Hence, it may play a major role in reducing appetite and resisting body fat, and thus helping to lose weight, so cinnamon can be deservedly considered one of the effective slimming herbs.

Side effects of cinnamon

Although the use of cinnamon may be safe, in some cases we must be careful and avoid regular and excessive use of it.

Excessive use of it may lead to a drop in blood pressure , and it may also pose a risk to the following:

Pregnant or breastfeeding women.
People who suffer from allergies to it.
Ginger for slimming
One of the herbs for weight loss is ginger , which is one of the healthy foods that is effective in losing weight.

The many health benefits of ginger are :
It contains a high percentage of fiber, which facilitates bowel movement and helps lower cholesterol levels in the blood.
It helps prevent stomach ulcers by promoting mucus secretion.

Improves and helps digestion; It contains enzymes that act as catalysts for proteins to secrete digestive enzymes and increase stomach acidity.

Ginger is used to prevent nausea, especially morning sickness in pregnant women.

It allows and helps blood vessels to expand, thus helping to improve blood circulation, and this can greatly enhance metabolism.

It has been found that people who eat ginger may lose up to 20% more fat than those who do not eat it.

Side effects of ginger

Although ginger is one of the effective herbs for weight loss, eating too much of it has a side effect , as it may cause the following:

Nausea.
Allergies.
Digestive system disorders.

Green tea for weight loss

Green tea has long been known   as the number one herb for weight loss, and this is not because it produces a lot of urine, as some people think. This is not related to burning and losing fat, but rather because:

Its role and effect in accelerating and enhancing metabolism and burning fat in the body.

It contains antioxidants that have been associated with increased metabolism and the ability to stimulate fat burning.

Its effectiveness in increasing metabolism, most likely due to caffeine and polyphenols found in tea leaves.

It contains substances called catechins, which are plant chemicals that affect the metabolism process.

Side effects of green tea

Although green tea is one of the common herbs for weight loss, it causes some side effects. It causes:

Dehydration, as it reduces water retention, is a diuretic and contains caffeine, which is why it may not be recommended for those suffering from dehydration or those with high blood pressure.

Diarrhea.

Nervousness.

Flax seeds for weight loss

Flax seeds contain a high amount of fiber and a low amount of carbohydrates, hence they are included among the herbs for slimming and weight loss and are included in weight loss plans.

While the fat content of flaxseeds is ultimately high, they are good fats for the body, which makes them an excellent choice for both health and weight loss.

Flax seeds are one of the herbs for weight loss that are beneficial in all of the following:

It contains a resinous substance, and when soaked in water and eaten, it helps fill the stomach, thus feeling full and reducing the amount of food eaten during the day.

It helps reduce the risk of heart disease , as it is a rich source of Omega-3, fatty acids, and useful fibers to enhance heart health, reduce blood pressure, and reduce bad cholesterol in the body.

Its peel contributes to fighting and preventing cancer.

Side effects of flax seeds

Although flax seeds are beneficial for weight loss, they may increase weight if consumed in large quantities. They are a double-edged sword, and flax seeds may also cause the following harms:

Allergies.

Digestive system disorders.

Ginseng to lose weight

Ginseng is a medicinal herb for weight loss that helps increase the body's energy secretion and stamina, thus fighting fatigue and exhaustion. Thus, it may help with the following:

Increase your rate of physical activity, which is necessary for weight loss.

Reducing blood sugar levels, thus helping to lose weight.

Contributing to the transfer of fats from the liver, so that the body can use them to obtain energy, increase metabolic rates in the body, and reduce the level of bad cholesterol in the blood.

Side effects of ginseng

Taking ginseng in large quantities may cause the following:

Sleep disorders and insomnia.

Allergies.

Turmeric to burn fat

Turmeric is famous   for its many benefits in treating many diseases and infections, and this may be due to the powerful antioxidants it contains, but what about it being a weight loss herb?

It has been found that turmeric has a good effect on weight loss, because it has the following benefits:

It stimulates the production of bile in the liver and its secretion through the gallbladder, which enhances digestion and metabolism.

Anti-inflammatory, especially gastrointestinal and respiratory infections.

Gas repellent.

Contributing to the treatment of some digestive system problems and intestinal problems, such as: diarrhea and irritable bowel syndrome.

Side effects of turmeric

Despite the benefits of turmeric, it harms the following groups:

Gallbladder patients.

People who suffer from allergies to it.

Important tips when using herbs for weight loss

Herbs for weight loss can help in losing weight, but at a rate that may be simple and not fast and clear, especially for people who suffer from excessive obesity, so the following tips should be followed when thinking about using them:

Use herbs for weight loss in the correct proportions and do not exceed them, as this is a double-edged sword.

Consult your doctor when starting to take any type of herb.

Follow a healthy lifestyle, and you must always realize that real and permanent weight loss is in a complete lifestyle change.

Stay away from some herbs for weight loss if you fall into the following categories:

People who suffer from high blood pressure and cholesterol.

Diabetics.

Kidney and liver patients.

Finally, we say, make every day a goal for you and do not focus on only the distant and final goals that may make you despair. Make every day and every minute a destination to focus on for the sake of change. This way, you will not lose your will and patience in the change that you aspire to, and every day will become a new day for the challenge. The balance between body, spirit and mind .

You can follow my account on Amazon to receive everything new from me And don't forget to read the second part of the series of alternative medicine books

Thank you for choosing the Alternative Medicine series of books.

I wish you a happy day

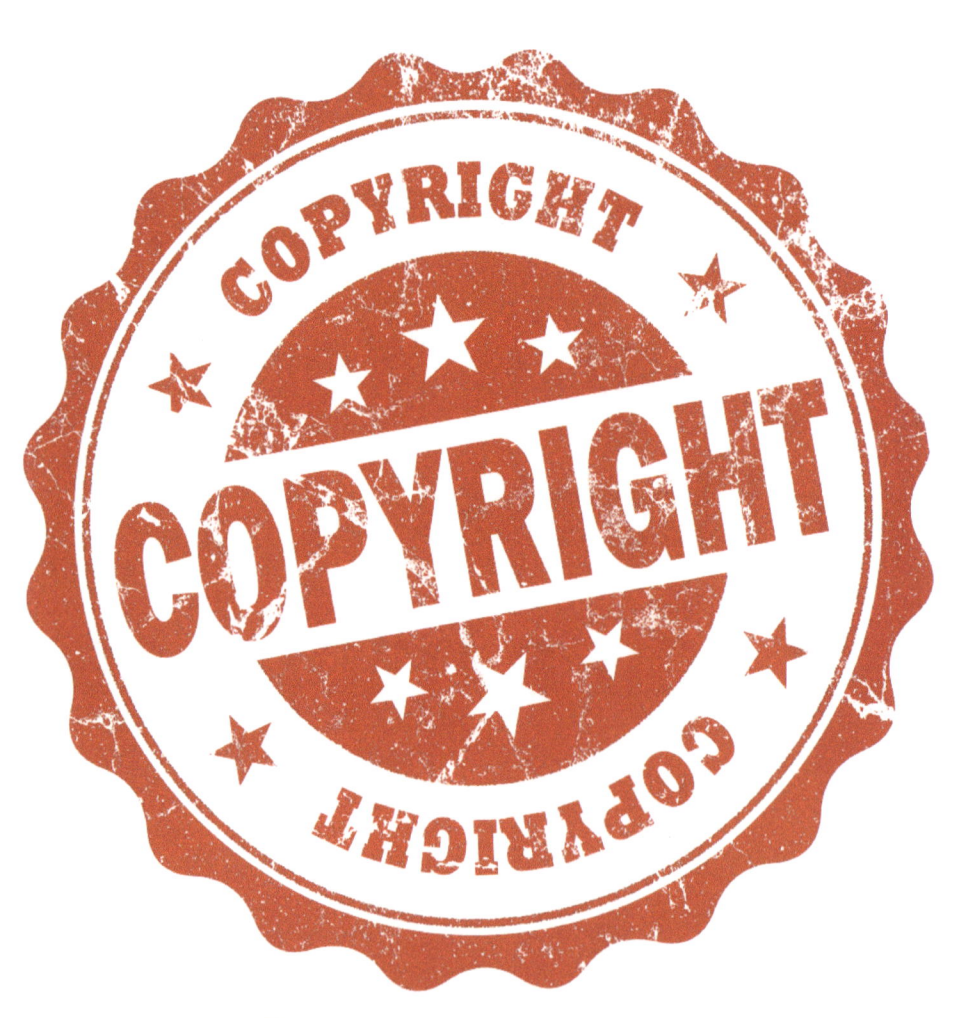